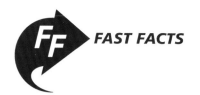

C000148042

Peripheral T-cell Lymphoma

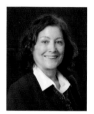

Francine M Foss MD
Professor of Medicine (Hematology) and of Dermatology
Yale University School of Medicine
New Haven, Connecticut, USA

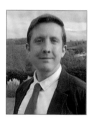

Matthew Ahearne MBChB MD MRCP FRCPath
Consultant Haematologist
University Hospitals of Leicester NHS Trust
Leicester, UK

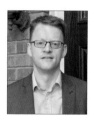

Christopher P Fox MBChB(Hons) MRCP FRCPath PhD
Consultant Haematologist
Nottingham University Hospitals NHS Foundation Trust
Nottingham, UK

Chapter 7 was written by Lohith Gowda MD MRCP (UK), Hematology and Bone
Marrow Transplantation, Yale University School of Medicine, New Haven, CT, USA.

Declaration of Independence
This book is as balanced and as practical as we can make it.
Ideas for improvement are always welcome: fastfacts@karger.com

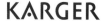

Fast Facts: Peripheral T-cell Lymphoma
First published 2019
Text © 2019 Francine M Foss, Matthew Ahearne and Christopher P Fox
© 2019 in this edition S. Karger Publishers Limited

S. Karger Publishers Limited, Elizabeth House, Queen Street, Abingdon, Oxford
OX14 3LN, UK. Tel: +44 (0)1235 523233

Book orders can be placed by telephone (+41 61 306 1440), email (orders@
karger.com) or via the website at: karger.com

Fast Facts is a trademark of S. Karger Publishers Limited.

A CIP record for this title is available from the British Library.

ISBN 978-1-912776-18-4

Foss F (Francine)
Fast Facts: Peripheral T-cell Lymphoma/
Francine M Foss, Matthew Ahearne, Christopher P Fox

Writing support for chapters 1, 2, and 3 from
Helen Barham PhD, The Text Doctor, Wantage, UK.

Typesetting by Thomas Bohm, User Design, Illustration
and Typesetting, UK.
Printed in the UK with Xpedient Print.

Made possible by a contribution from Takeda Pharmaceuticals Company
Limited. Takeda did not have any influence on the content and all items were
subject to independent peer and editorial review.

List of abbreviations

ALK: anaplastic lymphoma kinase

alloSCT: allogeneic stem cell transplantation

ASCT: autologous stem cell transplantation

BCL: B-cell lymphoma protein (BCL-2, BCL-6)

BCL-XL: B-cell lymphoma extra-large protein

CAR: chimeric antigen receptor

CAR T: chimeric antigen receptor T cell

CCR: CC chemokine receptor (CCR3, CCR4)

CD: cluster of differentiation

CIBMTR: Center for International Blood and Marrow Transplantation Registry

CNS: central nervous system

CR: complete response

CR1: first complete remission

CT: computed tomography

CTCL: cutaneous T-cell lymphoma

ctDNA: circulating tumor DNA

CTLA-4: cytotoxic T-lymphocyte-associated protein 4

CXCL: C-X-C motif chemokine ligand

CXCR: C-X-C motif chemokine receptor

DLBLC: diffuse large B-cell lymphoma

DOR: duration of response

EBER: Epstein–Barr virus encoding region

EBV: Epstein–Barr virus

EFS: event-free survival

EMA: epithelial membrane antigen

EOMES: eomesodermin

FDA: Food and Drug Administration

FDG: fluorodeoxyglucose

FoxP3: forkhead box P3 (scurfin)

GATA-3: GATA binding protein 3

GVHD: graft versus host disease

GVL: graft versus lymphoma

HDAC: histone deacetylase

HDT: high-dose chemotherapy

HLA: human leukocyte antigen

HTLV-1: human T lymphotropic virus

ICOS: inducible T-cell co-stimulator

IL: interleukin

iPET: interim positron emission tomography

IPI: International Prognostic Index

ISH: in situ hybridization

ITK: interleukin-2-inducible T-cell kinase

JAK: Janus kinase

Ki-67: a cellular marker for differentiation

KIR: killer inhibitory receptor

LDH: lactate dehydrogenase

LMP: latent protein membrane

MDR: multidrug resistance protein

MHC: major histocompatibility complex

MMAE: monomethyl auristatin E

MRI: magnetic resonance imaging

MUM1: multiple myeloma oncogene 1

NF-κB: nuclear factor kappa light-chain-enhancer of activated B cells

NGS: next-generation sequencing

NHL: non-Hodgkin lymphoma

NK: natural killer

NPM: nucleophosmin

NRM: non-relapse mortality

ORR: overall response rate

OS: overall survival

PAX5: paired box 5

PD1: programmed cell death receptor 1

PD-L1: programmed cell death ligand 1

PET: positron emission tomography

PFS: progression-free survival

PGP: P glycoprotein pump

PI3K: phosphatidyl-inositol 3-kinase

PLCG1: phospholipase C gamma 1

PR: partial response

PRDM1: PR domain zinc finger protein 1

PTCL: peripheral T-cell lymphoma

RIC: reduced-intensity conditioning

SAP: signaling lymphocytic activation molecule (SLAM)-associated protein

SEER: Surveillance, Epidemiology, and End Results

TBX21: T-box 21

TCR: T-cell receptor

TCRB: T-cell receptor beta chain

TCRG: T-cell receptor gamma chain

TdT: terminal deoxynucleotidyl transferase

Tfh: follicular helper T cell

TIA-1: a cytotoxic granule-associated protein

TRM: treatment-related mortality

WES: whole-exome sequencing

WGS: whole-genome sequencing

WHO: World Health Organization

Chemotherapy regimens

ABVD: Adriamycin (doxorubicin), bleomycin, vinblastine and dacarbazine

AspaMetDex: L-asparaginase, methotrexate and dexamethasone

BEAC: carmustine (BCNU), etoposide, cytarabine (Ara C) and cyclophosphamide

BEAM: carmustine (BCNU), etoposide, cytarabine (Ara C) and melphalan

CHOEP: CHOP and etoposide

CHOP: cyclophosphamide, hydroxydaunorubicin (doxorubicin), Oncovin (vincristine) and prednisolone

CHP + A: cyclophosphamide, hydroxydaunorubicin (doxorubicin), prednisolone and brentuximab vedotin (Adcetris)

DeVIC: dexamethasone, etoposide, ifosfamide and carboplatin

DHAP: dexamethasone, high-dose Ara C (cytarabine) and cisplatin

ESHAP: etoposide, methylprednisolone, high-dose Ara-C (cytarabine) and cisplatin

GDP: gemcitabine, dexamethasone and cisplatin

GELOX: gemcitabine, oxaliplatin and L-asparaginase

GemOx: gemcitabine and oxaliplatin

GEM-P: gemcitabine, cisplatin and methylprednisolone

GVD: gemcitabine, vinorelbine and pegylated liposomal doxorubicin

ICE: ifosfamide, carboplatin and etoposide

IVE: ifosfamide, epirubicin and etoposide

MAC: methotrexate/ leucovorin, actinomycin D and cyclophosphamide or chlorambucil

PEGS: cisplatin, etoposide, gemcitabine and methylprednisolone

SMILE: dexamethasone, methotrexate, ifosfamide, L-asparaginase and etoposide

VIP: etoposide, ifosfamide and cisplatin

Types of PTCL

The following abbreviations are used throughout this book.

AITL: angioimmunoblastic T-cell lymphoma

ALCL: anaplastic large-cell lymphoma

ATLL: adult T-cell leukemia/ lymphoma

EATL: enteropathy-associated T-cell lymphoma

ENKTCL: extranodal natural killer/ T-cell lymphoma

HSTCL: hepatosplenic T-cell lymphoma

MEITL: monomorphic epitheliotropic intestinal T-cell lymphoma

PTCL-NOS: peripheral T-cell lymphoma not otherwise specified

Tfh-related: follicular helper T cell-related

Introduction

The peripheral T-cell lymphomas (PTCL) are a heterogeneous group of rare entities, accounting for 10–15% of non-Hodgkin lymphomas. These lymphomas commonly arise in extranodal sites as well as in nodal tissue.

The classification of the PTCLs is evolving but is traditionally based on clinical presentation, encompassing nodal, extranodal and leukemic types. The accurate diagnosis of PTCL subtypes is challenging and requires careful integration of the clinical picture, morphology, immunohistochemistry, flow cytometry, cytogenetics and molecular biology.

By contrast with the B-cell lymphomas, we are only just beginning to develop individualized treatment algorithms based on PTCL subtype. First-line treatment with conventional chemotherapy is often not curative but patients in remission may proceed to consolidative stem cell transplantation, which may offer an increased chance of cure, or at least long-term disease control. Clinical and biological heterogeneity across the PTCL subtypes presents challenges in the design and conduct of potentially practice-changing comparative clinical trials, and, overall, the prognosis remains guarded for most patients.

Whilst the diagnosis and treatment of PTCL require specialist expertise, this new *Fast Facts* title provides an informative overview that will be useful to anyone involved in the care of patients with PTCL, including hematologists, oncologists, specialist nurses and primary care providers, as well as medical students. This resource raises awareness of these rare lymphomas and describes the current – and emerging – approaches to diagnosis and treatment.

1   T-cell biology

The immune system combats foreign pathogens through innate and acquired (or adaptive) immunity (Figure 1.1).

- Innate immunity offers a rapid but non-specific defense. It comprises the physical epithelial barrier, complement activation, some T cells and natural killer (NK) cells, and phagocytic cells (neutrophils and macrophages) which engulf and remove pathogens.
- In the adaptive immune system, T and B cells recognize and respond to specific antigens, producing a tailored response to invading pathogens. Persistence of these 'experienced' T and B cells results in long-term immune memory.

T cells

T cells develop from progenitors within the thymus gland. Mature T cells can be broadly classified into two types:

- T-helper cells, which are primarily involved in coordinating the immune response to an invading organism
- cytotoxic T cells, which kill cells infected with microorganisms.

T-cell receptors (TCRs) are analogous to the immunoglobulin molecules in B cells. Early T cells express TCRs in germline configuration. Recombination of TCR genes during maturation of T cells produces a unique TCR configuration – a critical feature of protective immunity that enables mature T cells to recognize and respond to a broad range of foreign material.

    TCRs comprise two different protein chains (i.e. they are heterodimers), most often an alpha and beta subunit ($\alpha\beta$ T cells). These $\alpha\beta$ T cells recognize and bind foreign peptides presented by major histocompatibility complex (MHC) molecules on the cell surface of antigen-presenting cells. This MHC–antigen complex binds to $\alpha\beta$ TCRs, while other co-stimulatory molecules (e.g. CD28) are activated, leading to $\alpha\beta$ T-cell activation, proliferation, differentiation and apoptosis and cytokine release.

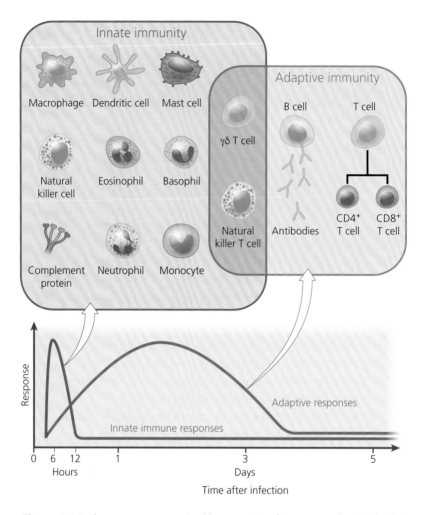

Figure 1.1 Pathogens are recognized by a variety of immune cells. The body's initial non-specific innate immunity is triggered in the first critical hours of exposure to a new pathogen. The adaptive immunity develops over several days in response to specific antigens.

About 5% of T cells express a gamma and delta TCR (γδ T cells). These cells have similarities with NK cells, with roles in both innate and adaptive immune responses.[1] They are typically found at sites of antigen contact, such as the skin, spleen, liver, intestine and bone marrow. As a first line of defense after antigenic stimulus, γδ T cells release cytotoxic factors (perforins, granzyme B and TIA-1). The γδ TCR is expressed by several extranodal subtypes of PTCL (see Chapter 2).

CD4 and CD8. Lymphoid progenitor cells in the thymus undergo stepwise maturation (Figure 1.2). The developing cells, called thymocytes, do not initially express CD4 or CD8 (described as double negative); expression of CD4 and CD8 is driven by positive signals received during development, resulting in double-positive thymocytes. Double-positive cells also encounter self-antigens and those that exhibit self-reactivity undergo negative selection. Finally, either CD4 or CD8 is downregulated, resulting in single-positive cells. The naive CD4+ and CD8+ T cells enter the peripheral circulation from the thymus.

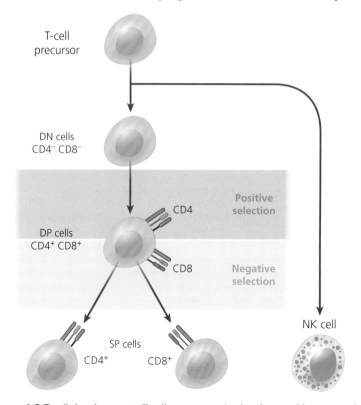

Figure 1.2 T-cell development. T-cell precursors in the thymus (thymocytes) develop into mature single-positive CD4+ or CD8+ cells. DN, double negative; DP, double positive; NK, natural killer; SP, single positive.

CD8+ T cells recognize antigens presented by the MHC class I molecules found on nucleated cells. Once activated, the CD8+ T cells proliferate to produce cytotoxic T lymphocytes – a population of effector T cells which release the enzymes and toxins that induce apoptosis.

CD4+ T cells recognize antigens presented by MHC class II molecules, which are only present on specialized antigen-presenting cells. Most of these cells are 'helper' subsets, which release cytokines, sending positive signals to other immune cells, predominantly B cells (Figure 1.3). A unique subset of CD4+ T cells, called T regulatory cells, restrain the immune response via various cytokine and signaling mechanisms, preventing aberrant or exaggerated immune activation.[2] Follicular helper T cells provide essential support for B-cell immune responses.[3]

Our understanding of T-cell subsets has advanced significantly over recent years. The external signals (cytokines) that trigger polarized T-cell differentiation are being elucidated, as are the molecular mechanisms that alter T-cell behavior to produce specific effector functions. Furthermore, gene expression profiling is being used to define the molecular signatures of T-cell subsets. These insights are refining our understanding of PTCL subtypes and have allowed the cell of origin to be identified for some (see Chapter 2).[4]

Natural killer cells

NK cells are a type of lymphocyte derived from the same common lymphoid progenitor as B and T lymphocytes but develop primarily in the bone marrow. NK cells are typically considered part of the innate immune system because they rapidly produce inflammatory cytokines and directly kill infected cells without prior priming or activation. However, recent evidence suggests that NK cells are also important in adaptive immunity.[5]

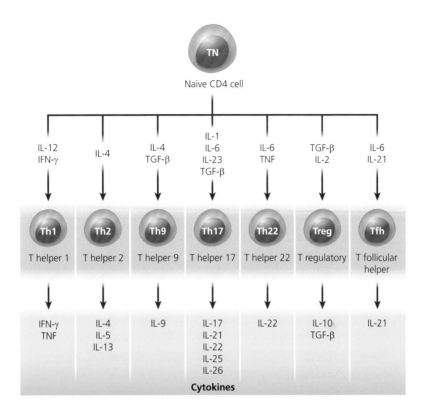

Figure 1.3 Differentiation of naive CD4 cells into helper T-cell subsets. CD4, cluster of differentiation; IFN, interferon; IL, interleukin; Tfh, follicular helper T cell; TGF, transforming growth factor; Th, helper T cell; TN, naive T cell; TNF, tumor necrosis factor; Treg, regulatory T cell.

Key points – T-cell biology

- T cells develop in the thymus and are part of the innate and adaptive immune system. They recognize and respond to specific antigens, producing a tailored response to invading pathogens.
- Mature T cells express a surface T-cell receptor (TCR) that recognizes fragments of antigen as peptides bound to major histocompatibility complex (MHC) molecules.
- Thymocytes do not express CD4 or CD8 initially (double-negative) but become double-positive during development, after which one molecule is downregulated. CD8⁺ T cells (cytotoxic T lymphocytes) recognize antigens presented by the MHC class I molecules found on nucleated cells. CD4⁺ T cells, of which there are several subtypes, recognize antigens presented by MHC class II molecules, which are only present on specialized antigen-presenting cells.
- Natural killer (NK) cells derive from the same common lymphoid progenitor as T cells but develop primarily in the bone marrow. They produce inflammatory cytokines and directly kill infected cells without prior priming or activation. While NK cells are typically considered part of the innate immune system, recent evidence suggests that they are also important in adaptive immunity.

Key references

1. Chien YH, Meyer C, Bonneville M. Gammadelta T cells: first line of defense and beyond. *Annu Rev Immunol* 2014;32:121–55.

2. Vignali DA, Collison LW, Workman CJ. How regulatory T cells work. *Nat Rev Immunol* 2008;8:523–32.

3. Crotty S. Follicular helper CD4 T cells (TFH). *Annu Rev Immunol* 2011;29:621–63.

4. Iqbal J, Wright G, Wang C et al. Gene expression signatures delineate biological and prognostic subgroups in peripheral T-cell lymphoma. *Blood* 2014;123:2915–23.

5. Moretta A, Marcenaro E, Parolini S et al. NK cells at the interface between innate and adaptive immunity. *Cell Death Differ* 2008;15:226–33.

Further reading

Clarke S, Li BT. Components of the immune system. In: *Fast Facts: Immuno-Oncology*. S. Karger Publishers Limited, 2017:11–23.

2 Classification

Lymphomas arise from a single abnormal lymphocyte. Genetic changes within this lymphocyte lead to an accumulation of identical cells, known as a clonal population. The genetic changes that give rise to a clonal population may arise during different stages of the cell life cycle, which is important in classification.

To date, the classification of T-cell lymphomas has been based largely on morphologic assessment, which contrasts with the B-cell lymphomas, for which certain entities are defined by distinct immunophenotypic profiles corresponding to specific maturation stages and recurrent chromosomal translocations.

The classification of PTCLs is complicated by the diversity of the entities, a relative lack of pathognomonic molecular markers, and overlapping clinical and pathological features. Multiple genetic aberrations have been identified in T-cell lymphomas but few are entity defining. Two distinct subsets have been identified that span multiple histopathological groups:[1]

- T-cell lymphomas arising from follicular helper T cells (Tfh) – angioimmunoblastic T-cell lymphoma (AITL), Tfh subtype of PTCL not otherwise specified (NOS), Tfh T-cell lymphoma
- γδ T-cell lymphomas – primary cutaneous γδ T-cell lymphoma, hepatosplenic T-cell lymphoma (HSTCL).

There is also evidence of plasticity in terms of cellular derivation (αβ, γδ, natural killer [NK]), particularly in the extranodal entities with a cytotoxic profile.

WHO classification

The World Health Organization (WHO) classification of hematopoietic and lymphoid tumors divides PTCLs into nodal, extranodal and leukemic types, each with multiple disease entities (Table 2.1).[2] The 2016 update incorporated advances in understanding of the cell of origin and the molecular signatures of particular types of PTCL (Table 2.2).[3]

TABLE 2.1

Key types of PTCL based on the World Health Organization classification[2]

Nodal	PTCL not otherwise specified (PTCL-NOS)
	Anaplastic large-cell lymphoma (ALCL) which may be ALK$^+$ or ALK$^-$
	Angioimmunoblastic T-cell lymphoma (AITL)
Extranodal	Pleiomorphic enteropathy-associated T-cell lymphoma (EATL)
	Monomorphic epitheliotropic intestinal T-cell lymphoma (MEITL, formerly EATL type 2)
	Extranodal natural killer/T-cell lymphoma (ENKTCL)
	Hepatosplenic T-cell lymphoma (HSTCL)
	Panniculitis-like T-cell lymphoma ($\alpha\beta$ subtype)
Leukemic	Adult T-cell leukemia/lymphoma (ATLL) associated with HTLV-1
	T-cell prolymphocytic leukemia
	Large granular lymphocytic leukemia
	Aggressive NK-cell leukemia

ALK, anaplastic lymphoma kinase; HTLV-1, human T-cell lymphotropic virus 1; NK, natural killer.

PTCL not otherwise specified

PTCL-NOS refers to subtypes of PTCL that do not fit into the distinct entities described in this chapter and is in fact the most common category, accounting for 30–35% of cases of PTCL. This largely reflects the need to more precisely characterize these lymphomas.

PTCL-NOS are predominantly considered to be nodal lymphomas, although extranodal involvement at presentation or relapse is common. The most common extranodal sites are the skin and gastrointestinal tract but the bone marrow, lungs and peripheral blood may also be involved.

TABLE 2.2

Characteristics of PTCL subtypes

Type of T-cell lymphoma	Immunophenotypic features		TCR	Cell of origin
	Cluster of differentiation (CD)	Others		
Nodal				
PTCL-NOS	CD4 > CD8 CD5↓⁻, CD7↓/⁻ CD30⁺/⁻ CD56⁺/⁻	Subset with Tfh features, CG⁺/⁻	αβ, rarely γδ	Mostly Th, but varies
AITL	CD4⁺ CD10⁺/⁻	BCL6⁺/⁻, CXCL13⁺ PD1⁺, ICOS⁺ SAP⁺/⁻, CCR5⁺/⁻ hyperplasia of FDC EBV⁺ B blasts	αβ	Tfh
ALCL ALK⁺/⁻	CD4⁺/⁻ CD3⁺/⁻, CD25⁺ CD30⁺	EMA⁺, CG⁺	αβ	CTL
Extranodal				
EATL	CD8⁽⁺⁾/⁻ CD56⁻	HLA-DQ2/8	αβ	IE T cells, pre-existing enteropathy
MEITL	CD8⁺ CD56⁺		γδ or αβ	IE T cells or NK, no pre-existing enteropathy
ENKTCL	CD3⁺/⁻,* CD56⁺ CD8⁺/⁻	Granzyme B⁺ TIA-1⁺, perforin⁺ EBER⁺, LMP1	Germline configuration, rarely αβ or γδ	NK, less commonly CTL
HSTCL	CD4⁻, CD8⁺/⁻ CD3⁺, CD5⁻ CD56⁺/⁻	TIA-1⁺ granzyme M⁺ granzyme B⁻ perforin⁻	γδ, rarely αβ	CTL

*Surface CD3⁻, cytoplasmic CD3ε⁺.
↓ reduced (not absent) levels; ALK, anaplastic lymphoma kinase; CG, cytotoxic granules;
CTL, cytotoxic T lymphocyte; EBV, Epstein–Barr virus; FDC, follicular dendritic cell;
HLA, human leukocyte antigen; IE, intraepithelial; NK, natural killer; TCR, T-cell receptor;
Tfh, follicular helper T cell; Th, T helper cell. Cell markers are defined in the list of
abbreviations (page 4). Adapted from d'Amore et al. 2015.[3]

Morphology. Involvement at a node is often diffuse but can be interfollicular or paracortical, obscuring the normal architecture of the node; the number of high endothelial venules (post-capillary venous swellings where lymphocytes enter a lymph node from the blood) is also increased. Extensive immunophenotyping may be required to distinguish PTCL-NOS from AITL. The cytology in PTCL-NOS is often pleomorphic (Figure 2.1) – most cases comprise a mixed population of medium to large cells with a high proliferation rate. Clear cells are frequently present.

Immunophenotypic features. The expression of pan T-cell antigens (i.e. those found on all T cells) by malignant cells is highly variable in PTCL-NOS, with reduced or no expression of CD5 and CD7 in up to 80% of cases. Loss of CD3 and CD2 expression is less common. The predominant immunophenotype in PTCL-NOS is CD3+, CD4+, with no cytotoxic markers. However, a subset expresses CD8 with cytotoxic markers (TIA-1, granzyme B and perforin) and CD56, and other subsets can show double positivity or double negativity for CD4 and CD8. The expression of CD52 varies widely (35–100%), and 32–58% of PTCL-NOS cases express CD30 (an activation marker for B and T cells). CD30 positivity is typically focal but with variable staining intensity,

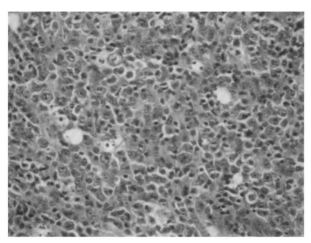

Figure 2.1 PTCL not otherwise specified: inguinal lymph node showing effacement with small and medium size pleomorphic T-cell infiltrate.

and thus can be difficult to distinguish from anaplastic lymphoma kinase (ALK)⁻ anaplastic large-cell lymphoma (ALCL).

Molecular characteristics. The 2016 update to the WHO classification reassigned several entities formerly listed under PTCL-NOS, based on genetic analyses. Two major prognostic subgroups of PTCL-NOS have recently been identified based on overexpression of:
- GATA-3 and its target genes (*CCR4*, *IL18RA*, *CXCR7*, *IK*), which play key roles in regulating T helper cell 2 differentiation
- TBX21 and EOMES and their target genes (*CXCR3*, *IL2RB*, *CCL3*, *IFNγ*) which regulate T helper cell 1 differentiation.

TCR gene rearrangements are often present in PTCL-NOS, with more than 85% expressing αβ-TCR and fewer expressing γδ-TCR or being TCR-silent.[4] *PDGFRA* and activated *NOTCH1* are often overexpressed in PTCL-NOS.

Anaplastic large-cell lymphoma

Morphology. Histologically, ALCL is characterized by sheets of pleomorphic cells, typically large anaplastic cells with abundant cytoplasm, vesicular chromatin and variably prominent nucleoli (Figure 2.2). Some have a kidney bean or horseshoe-shaped nucleus, termed 'hallmark' cells, or multiple nuclei that form a peripheral wreathlike configuration along the cytoplasmic membrane ('wreath' cells). The markedly atypical malignant cells occasionally resemble Reed–Sternberg cells. Nuclear cytoplasmic invaginations (pseudoinclusions) may also be seen, termed 'doughnut' cells.

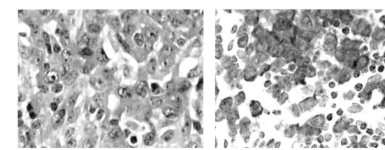

Figure 2.2 Anaplastic large-cell lymphoma (ALCL): (a) hematoxylin and eosin stain, showing infiltration by anaplastic lymphoid cells; (b) immunostain for anaplastic lymphoma kinase.

Additional (variant) morphologic patterns may be seen in ALK[+] ALCL, including:

- small cell (5–10%), with small to intermediate sized, often perivascular, cells
- lymphohistiocytic (10%), with a mixture of histiocytes
- Hodgkin-like (< 5%), with a nodular sclerosing background.

More than one pattern may be seen.

Immunophenotypic features. ALCL is a CD4[+] T-cell lymphoma (although rare CD8[+] cases have been reported), characterized by strong and robust expression of CD30 in the cell membrane and Golgi bodies, particularly in the larger cells.

Expression of other T-cell markers varies widely between patients. ALK[+] ALCL most commonly expresses CD2 and CD5, whereas ALK[-] ALCL most commonly expresses CD2 and CD3. Expression of EMA and CD45 varies widely and is more common in ALK[+] ALCL. Cytotoxic markers and CD43 are expressed in most cases but may be absent from ALK[-] ALCL with *DUSP22–IRF4* rearrangement.[5,6] MUM1 is consistently expressed, and dot-like clustering may be seen in the cytoplasm – a possible differentiator from PTCL-NOS. ALCLs are negative for PAX5, Epstein–Barr virus (EBV), CD56 and CD15, although some cases with variable CD15 and CD56 expression have been reported. Expression of ALK in ALK[+] ALCL is usually nuclear and cytoplasmic, characteristic of the *NPM1–ALK* translocation (> 80% of cases) or diffuse cytoplasmic with peripheral prominence (TPM3–ALK; 10% of cases).

Molecular characteristics. Most patients with ALK[+] ALCL (60–70%) have a translocation between chromosomes 2 and 5, such that the ALK gene portion on chromosome 2 that codes for the tyrosine kinase comes under the control of the nucleophosmin (NPM) promotor on chromosome 5, resulting in permanent expression of a chimeric NPM–ALK protein. This is an aberrant tyrosine kinase, and is thought to trigger malignant transformation via constitutive phosphorylation of intracellular targets. Less common ALK fusion proteins associated with ALCL result from t(1;2), t(2;3), inv(2) and t(2;22) translocations. In all cases, the ALK tyrosine kinase domain becomes linked to an alternative promotor that regulates its expression.

ALK⁺ and ALK⁻ ALCLs have been reported to have different gene expression profiles.[7]

- *BCL6*, *PTPN12*, *CEBPB* and *SERPINA1* are preferentially overexpressed in ALK⁺ ALCL.
- *CCR7*, *CNTFR* and *IL22* are preferentially overexpressed in ALK⁻ ALCL.

Chromosomal rearrangements of *DUSP22* and *TP63* genes have recently been found in 30% and 8% of ALK⁻ ALCLs, respectively, but are absent from ALK⁺ ALCLs. Survival appears to be more favorable for patients with the *DUSP22* mutation but is poor for those with the *TP63* mutation, and intermediate for patients with ALK⁻ ALCL that lacks either rearrangement.[8]

Breast implant-associated ALCL, first described in 1997, is a rare and distinct clinicopathological entity in the most recent WHO classification (provisional status). It typically presents with seroma around the implant, and tumor cells are found within the capsule. It may be associated with specific bacterial pathogens[9] and with irregular- rather than smooth-surfaced implants.

Angioimmunoblastic T-cell lymphoma

AITL was originally considered to be a dysregulated immune response, but clonality studies have established it as a malignant lymphoma. Gene expression studies show a similar gene expression pattern to Tfh cells, a distinct CD4⁺ T-cell subset, suggesting that this is the cell of origin in AITL.[10,11] Normal Tfh cells provide essential support for B-cell immune responses; this explains why many of the distinct clinicopathological features of AITL reflect immune activation.

Morphology. Lymph node biopsies typically show a heavy stromal infiltrate comprising plasma cells, histiocytes, eosinophils and immunoblasts (Figure 2.3). Malignant T cells may represent only a minor component of the infiltrate, so accurate diagnosis can be challenging. Follicular dendritic cell networks are often expanded, and blood vessels typically demonstrate an unusual arborizing (tree-like branching) pattern.

The morphology of AITL can overlap with reactive entities and other lymphoid malignancies such as classic Hodgkin lymphoma

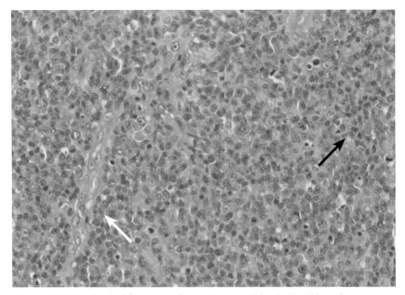

Figure 2.3 Histological features of angioimmunoblastic T-cell lymphoma: hematoxylin and eosin stain of an affected lymph node showing a pleomorphic infiltrate of lymphocytes throughout, prominent numbers of eosinophils (black arrow) and expanded vascularization (white arrow).

and T-cell-rich large B-cell lymphoma. B cells infected with EBV may resemble Reed–Sternberg cells, potentially causing confusion with classic Hodgkin lymphoma (Figure 2.4).

Immunophenotypic features. The malignant T cells in AITL typically express normal Tfh cell markers (CD10, BCL6, PD1, ICOS, CXCL13) and can be highlighted in tissue biopsies using immunohistochemistry antibodies. Individually, these markers are not specific for Tfh cells, as they are expressed on other T-cell subsets, but co-expression of two or three of these markers allows reliable identification of malignant Tfh cells.

Molecular characteristics. Molecular studies of AITL have demonstrated a unique mutational landscape. Mutations in the *TET2*, *DNMT3A* and *IDH2* epigenetic modifiers are typically associated with myeloid cancers but are also common in AITL; *TET2* and *DNMT3A* mutations may occur within hematopoietic stem cells.

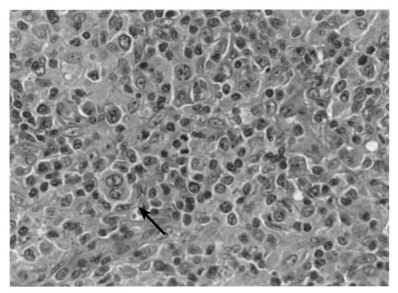

Figure 2.4 Activated B cells, usually Epstein–Barr virus positive, found within angioimmunoblastic T-cell lymphoma may resemble Reed–Sternberg cells, making differentiation from Hodgkin lymphoma difficult.

A recurrent hotspot mutation in the gene *RHOA* (*RHOA*^{G17V}) has been reported in 50–70% of AITL cases, although the exact function of this mutation has yet to be elucidated. Mutations in important genes involved in TCR signaling (*CD28*, *PLCG1*, *FYN*) have also been found.[12–16] Although TCR-related genes are mutated individually at relatively low frequencies across AITL cases (1–15%), up to half of all AITL harbor at least one TCR mutation.

Other follicular T cell-related lymphomas
Recent studies have shown that other PTCL subtypes are also derived from Tfh cells (Figure 2.5).

Nodal PTCL with Tfh phenotype. The molecular signature of Tfh cells is found in about 20% of PTCL-NOS cases, suggesting an overlapping relationship with AITL. Although these cases do not meet the full clinicopathological criteria of AITL, they have some histological findings in common with AITL, express Tfh cell markers and have a similar mutational profile to AITL.

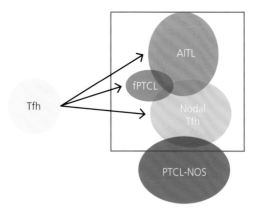

Figure 2.5 Distinct clinicopathological entities that share a follicular helper T-cell (Tfh) origin, suggesting a biologically distinct group from other PTCL entities. AITL, angioimmunoblastic T-cell lymphoma; fPTCL, follicular PTCL; NOS, not otherwise specified.

Follicular PTCL is a rare subtype with a follicular infiltrate of malignant T cells (Figure 2.6).[17,18] Previously considered a morphologic variant of PTCL-NOS, follicular PTCL is now understood to derive from Tfh cells based on a similar gene expression profile. Twenty percent of cases exhibit a t(5;9)(q33;q22) translocation that produces an *ITK–SYK* fusion gene, which acts as an oncogenic driver by mimicking the TCR signal.[19]

Intestinal PTCLs

Intestinal PTCLs are usually highly aggressive lymphomas of intraepithelial T cells and can be divided into two distinct forms:
- pleomorphic enteropathy-associated T-cell lymphoma (EATL)
- monomorphic epitheliotropic intestinal T-cell lymphoma (MEITL, formerly EATL type 2).

EATL occurs in the presence of gluten enteropathy, typically on a background of treatment-refractory celiac disease, although it occasionally presents de novo. Biopsies typically show features of active celiac disease in addition to infiltrative tumor (Figure 2.7). Tumor cells usually express αβ-TCR, lack CD4 and CD8 expression and are negative for CD56. CD30 is often expressed.[20]

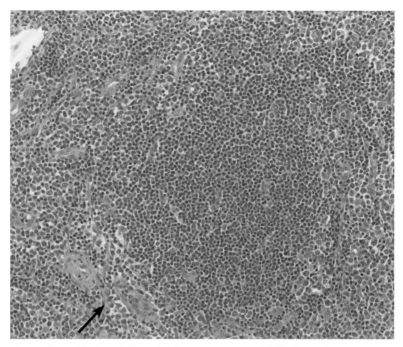

Figure 2.6 Follicular PTCL node showing preserved follicular architecture and prominent blood vessels (arrow).

MEITL is not associated with enteropathy or celiac disease and displays a distinct immunophenotype from EATL.[21] Tumor cells are typically positive for both CD8 and CD56, and most express γδ-TCR. The malignant infiltrate is monomorphic without the typical inflammatory background seen in EATL.

Molecular characteristics. Only a relatively small number of EATL and MEITL cases have been robustly characterized at the molecular level, and data relating to the molecular relationship of these two entities are conflicting, with some studies suggesting significant overlap while others report distinct profiles. Mutations in *SETD2*, *KRAS* and *STAT5B* appear to be more common in MEITL (*SETD2* and *STAT5B* mutations are more frequent in PTCL subtypes that express γδ-TCR, which explains the higher frequency in MEITL).[22] Mutations in *JAK-STAT* genes are frequent in both types.

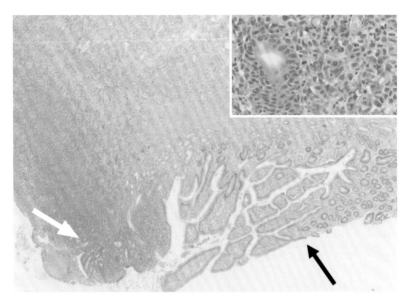

Figure 2.7 Enteropathy-associated T-cell lymphoma, showing an area of preserved villous architecture (black arrow) with an adjacent area exhibiting villous atrophy and tumor infiltrate (white arrow). The high-powered view (inset) highlights a diffuse population of atypical lymphoid cells. Image courtesy of Dr Hala Rashed, University Hospitals of Leicester.

Indolent T-cell lymphoproliferative disorder of the gastrointestinal tract is extremely rare. Biopsy demonstrates a dense, superficial lymphoid infiltrate with no significant epitheliotropism. It usually expresses CD8, although CD4 and NK cell markers may be seen rarely. Whilst clonal in nature, the proliferation fraction is typically less than 10%. It is essential that this indolent disorder, although rare, is not misdiagnosed as EATL or MEITL, because careful clinical follow-up alone may be sufficient.

Extranodal NK/T-cell lymphoma

The evolving lymphoma classification systems did not include extranodal natural killer/T cell lymphoma (ENKTCL) as a distinct entity because of early challenges in morphologic and phenotypic characterization. The Revised European–American Classification of Lymphoid Neoplasms used the term 'angiocentric lymphoma', but it is now recognized that this pathological description is not unique to ENKTCL. Other historic terminology included 'lethal midline granuloma' and 'rhinitis gangrenosa progressiva'. The recognition of ENKTCL as a unique clinicopathological entity that is strongly associated with EBV led to its formal incorporation into the WHO classification in 1999.

Morphology. Cytologically, the malignant NK/T cells appear as medium-sized lymphoid cells with pale cytoplasm containing azurophilic granules. The histology shows a pleomorphic infiltrate with evidence of angioinvasion and necrosis.

Immunophenotypic features. The characteristic phenotype of ENKTCL comprises CD2$^+$, CD56$^+$, surface CD3$^-$ (as demonstrated on fresh/frozen tissue) and cytoplasmic CD3ε^+ (demonstrated on formalin-fixed paraffin-embedded tissues), whilst a minority of ENKTCL cases display a cytotoxic CD8$^+$ T-cell phenotype. Importantly, all cases of ENKTCL display strong expression of EBV-encoded RNAs (EBER), such that the absence of EBER from tumor cells is highly suggestive of an alternative diagnosis. Immunostaining for the EBV latent membrane protein LMP1 is less sensitive than EBER for the detection of ENKTCL as this protein is expressed in only a subpopulation of ENKTCL cells.[23]

Molecular characteristics. Most cases originate from NK cells (see page 14) and have germline TCR gene configurations, whilst a proportion have clonal TCR rearrangements, in keeping with the phenotypic data.

Biopsy specimens from patients with ENKTCL are often small and necrotic, and repeated biopsy is often required for diagnosis; the availability of fresh tissue for molecular genetic studies is therefore limited. Disease-defining translocation events have not yet been confirmed, although genetic complexity is common.

Deletions of the long arm of chromosome 6 are seen with both conventional karyotyping and comparative genomic hybridization, indicating that tumor suppressor genes in these regions are involved in the pathogenesis of ENKTCL. The clonal form of EBV in ENKTCL cells, together with the expression of EBV-encoded transcripts and oncogenic proteins (LMP1 and LMP2), strongly suggests that lymphomagenesis is caused by EBV.

Hepatosplenic T-cell lymphoma

HSTCL is a rare variant of extranodal PTCL that may be associated with inflammatory bowel disease treated with multiple immunosuppressants.

Histological features. Significant sinusoidal infiltration in the liver, spleen and bone marrow with medium-sized cytotoxic T cells is a typical feature (Figure 2.8).

Morphology. HSTCL tissue demonstrates clusters of medium-sized monomorphic T cells with a loose rim of condensed chromatin, inconspicuous nucleoli, a pale cytoplasm and an indistinct cell membrane.

Immunophenotypic features. The typical phenotype is CD2⁺, CD3⁺, CD4⁻, CD5⁻, CD7⁺, CD8⁻, although CD8⁺ cases have been identified. The γδ phenotype can be elucidated on flow cytometry, with a characteristic absence of βF1 staining (directed against the β chain of αβ T cells).[24]

Molecular characteristics. Trisomy 8 and isochromosome 7q are the most common cytogenetic abnormalities in HSTCL.[25] Gene expression profiling has shown overexpression of NK markers such as KIR and the killer lectin-like receptors CD16, CD56 and NKG2F.[26] Oncogenes

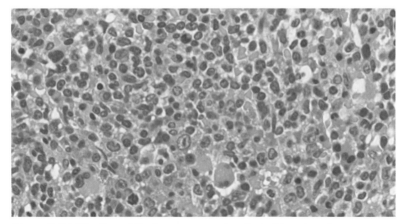

Figure 2.8 Infiltration of the bone marrow by atypical lymphocytes in hepatosplenic T-cell lymphoma (hematoxylin and eosin stain).

(*FOS, VA3*), cell trafficking-sphingosine phosphatase receptor-5 and the Syk kinase are also seen.[27] Mutations of epigenetic modifier genes such as *SETD2, INO80* and *ARID 1B* (62%) are found, as well as mutations in *STAT3* (9%), *STAT5B* (31%) and *PIK3CD* (9%).[28,29]

Adult T-cell leukemia/lymphoma

ATLL is a distinct subtype of PTCL, caused by human T-cell lymphotropic virus 1 (HTLV-1). It is relatively common in areas where HTLV-1 is endemic (south-west Japan, west Africa, the Caribbean, Brazil). Four clinical subtypes have been defined – acute, lymphoma, chronic and smoldering – based on the presence/absence of leukemic changes, high lactate dehydrogenase levels, hypercalcemia and organ infiltration; these subtypes inform the treatment strategy.

Morphology. The neoplastic cells are multilobulated with remarkable pleomorphism, often called 'flower cells' and may be seen in the peripheral blood (Figure 2.9).

Immunophenotypic features. The neoplastic cells express pan T-cell antigens but usually lack CD7, and most cases are CD4+. CD25 is usually strongly expressed whereas neoplastic cells are negative for ALK and cytotoxic markers. CD30 can be expressed, particularly in transformed cases. Neoplastic cells express FoxP3 and CD25, indicating peripheral CD4+ T regulatory cells as the cell of origin.[30]

Molecular characteristics. Genomic alterations in ATLL cluster tightly in genes associated with TCR NF-κB signaling, such as *PLCG1*, *PKC* and *CARD11*, and gain-of-function mutations have been identified in

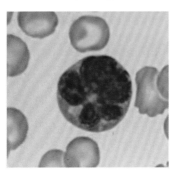

Figure 2.9 Human T-cell lymphotropic virus 1-associated T-cell leukemia: a malignant T lymphocyte showing a hyperconvoluted clover-leaf-like nucleus.

CCR4 and *CCR7*.[31] Another study has shown that the 3' region of the PD-L1 gene is disrupted by structural variations in 27% of ATLL cases, markedly increasing the number of aberrant PD-L1 transcripts.[32]

Key points – classification

- The PTCLs are a group of highly heterogeneous aggressive malignancies that arise from the transformation of mature post-thymic T cells and natural killer cells.
- The World Health Organization (WHO) classifies PTCLs into nodal, extranodal and leukemia types, each with multiple disease entities.
- PTCL not otherwise specified (PTCL-NOS) is the most common subtype, reflecting the need for more precise characterization of these lymphomas. Genetic analyses are helping to refine this category further.
- The primary nodal PTCLs are anaplastic large-cell lymphoma (ALCL), which may be positive or negative for the fusion protein anaplastic lymphoma kinase (ALK+/ALK−), and angioimmunoblastic T-cell lymphoma (AITL).
- Extranodal PTCLs are less common than nodal PTCLs and include enteropathy-associated T-cell lymphoma (EATL), NK/T-cell lymphoma (ENKTCL) and hepatosplenic T-cell lymphoma (HSTCL).
- Classification has been largely based on morphologic assessment, although the 2016 update to the WHO classification incorporated recent advances in the understanding of the cell of origin and the molecular signatures of particular types of PTCL. Genetic lesions are also being identified but few are entity-defining markers.

Key references

1. Gaulard P, de Leval L. Pathology of peripheral T-cell lymphomas: where do we stand? *Semin Hematol* 2014;51:5–16.

2. Campo E, Swerdlow SH, Harris NL et al. The 2008 WHO classification of lymphoid neoplasms and beyond: evolving concepts and practical applications. *Blood* 2011;117:5019–32.

3. d'Amore F, Gaulard P, Trumper L et al. Peripheral T-cell lymphomas: ESMO Clinical Practice Guidelines for diagnosis, treatment and follow-up. *Ann Oncol* 2015;26 Suppl 5:v108–15.

4. Piccaluga PP, Fuligni F, De Leo A et al. Molecular profiling improves classification and prognostication of nodal peripheral T-cell lymphomas: results of a phase III diagnostic accuracy study. *J Clin Oncol* 2013;31:3019–25.

5. King RL, Dao LN, McPhail ED et al. Morphologic features of ALK-negative anaplastic large cell lymphomas with DUSP22 rearrangements. *Am J Surg Pathol* 2016;40:36–43.

6. Xing X, Feldman AL. Anaplastic large cell lymphomas: ALK positive, ALK negative, and primary cutaneous. *Adv Anat Pathol* 2015;22:29–49.

7. Salaverria I, Bea S, Lopez-Guillermo A et al. Genomic profiling reveals different genetic aberrations in systemic ALK-positive and ALK-negative anaplastic large cell lymphomas. *Br J Haematol* 2008;140:516–26.

8. Parrilla Castellar ER, Jaffe ES, Said JW et al. ALK-negative anaplastic large cell lymphoma is a genetically heterogeneous disease with widely disparate clinical outcomes. *Blood* 2014;124:1473–80.

9. Miranda RN, Aladily TN, Prince HM et al. Breast implant-associated anaplastic large-cell lymphoma: long-term follow-up of 60 patients. *J Clin Oncol* 2014;32:114–20.

10. de Leval L, Rickman DS, Thielen C et al. The gene expression profile of nodal peripheral T-cell lymphoma demonstrates a molecular link between angioimmunoblastic T-cell lymphoma (AITL) and follicular helper T (TFH) cells. *Blood* 2007;109:4952–63.

11. Dupuis J, Boye K, Martin N et al. Expression of CXCL13 by neoplastic cells in angioimmunoblastic T-cell lymphoma (AITL): a new diagnostic marker providing evidence that AITL derives from follicular helper T cells. *Am J Surg Pathol* 2006;30:490–4.

12. Yoo HY, Sung MK, Lee SH et al. A recurrent inactivating mutation in RHOA GTPase in angioimmunoblastic T cell lymphoma. *Nat Genet* 2014;46:371–5.

13. Palomero T, Couronne L, Khiabanian H et al. Recurrent mutations in epigenetic regulators, RHOA and FYN kinase in peripheral T cell lymphomas. *Nat Genet* 2014;46:166–70.

14. Rohr J, Guo S, Huo J et al. Recurrent activating mutations of CD28 in peripheral T-cell lymphomas. *Leukemia* 2016;30: 1062–70.

15. Vallois D, Dobay MP, Morin RD et al. Activating mutations in genes related to TCR signaling in angioimmunoblastic and other follicular helper T-cell-derived lymphomas. *Blood* 2016;128: 1490–502.

16. Manso R, Rodriguez-Pinilla SM, Gonzalez-Rincon J et al. Recurrent presence of the PLCG1 S345F mutation in nodal peripheral T-cell lymphomas. *Haematologica* 2015;100:e25–7.

17. Agostinelli C, Hartmann S, Klapper W et al. Peripheral T cell lymphomas with follicular T helper phenotype: a new basket or a distinct entity? Revising Karl Lennert's personal archive. *Histopathology* 2011;59:679–91.

18. Miyoshi H, Sato K, Niino D et al. Clinicopathologic analysis of peripheral T-cell lymphoma, follicular variant, and comparison with angioimmunoblastic T-cell lymphoma: Bcl-6 expression might affect progression between these disorders. *Am J Clin Pathol* 2012;137:879–89.

19. Liang PI, Chang ST, Lin MY et al. Angioimmunoblastic T-cell lymphoma in Taiwan shows a frequent gain of ITK gene. *Int J Clin Exp Pathol* 2014;7:6097–107.

20. Wilson AL, Swerdlow SH, Przybylski GK et al. Intestinal gammadelta T-cell lymphomas are most frequently of type II enteropathy-associated T-cell type. *Hum Pathol* 2013;44:1131–45.

21. de Mascarel A, Belleannee G, Stanislas S et al. Mucosal intraepithelial T-lymphocytes in refractory celiac disease: a neoplastic population with a variable CD8 phenotype. *Am J Surg Pathol* 2008;32:744–51.

22. Nairismagi ML, Tan J, Lim JQ et al. JAK-STAT and G-protein-coupled receptor signaling pathways are frequently altered in epitheliotropic intestinal T-cell lymphoma. *Leukemia* 2016;30:1311–19.

23. Chiang AK, Tao Q, Srivastava G, Ho FC. Nasal NK- and T-cell lymphomas share the same type of Epstein–Barr virus latency as nasopharyngeal carcinoma and Hodgkin's disease. *Int J Cancer* 1996;68:285–90.

24. Gaulard P, Belhadj K, Reyes F. Gammadelta T-cell lymphomas. *Semin Hematol* 2003;40:233–43.

25. Kotlyar DS, Osterman MT, Diamond RH et al. A systematic review of factors that contribute to hepatosplenic T-cell lymphoma in patients with inflammatory bowel disease. *Clin Gastroenterol Hepatol* 2011;9:36–41 e1.

26. Miyazaki K, Yamaguchi M, Imai H et al. Gene expression profiling of peripheral T-cell lymphoma including gammadelta T-cell lymphoma. *Blood* 2009;113:1071–4.

27. Travert M, Huang Y, de Leval L et al. Molecular features of hepatosplenic T-cell lymphoma unravels potential novel therapeutic targets. *Blood* 2012;119:5795–806.

28. Nicolae A, Xi L, Pittaluga S et al. Frequent STAT5B mutations in γδ hepatosplenic T-cell lymphomas. *Leukemia* 2014;28: 2244–8.

29. McKinney M, Moffitt AB, Gaulard P et al. The genetic basis of hepatosplenic T-cell lymphoma. *Cancer Discov* 2017;7:369–79.

30. Karube K, Ohshima K, Tsuchiya T et al. Expression of FoxP3, a key molecule in CD4CD25 regulatory T cells, in adult T-cell leukaemia/lymphoma cells. *Br J Haematol* 2004;126:81–4.

31. Kataoka K, Nagata Y, Kitanaka A et al. Integrated molecular analysis of adult T cell leukemia/lymphoma. *Nat Genet* 2015;47:1304–15.

32. Kataoka K, Shiraishi Y, Takeda Y et al. Aberrant PD-L1 expression through 3'-UTR disruption in multiple cancers. *Nature* 2016;534:402–6.

3 Epidemiology and etiology

Incidence

T-cell lymphomas account for 10–15% of lymphoid malignancies, although the incidence varies geographically (see page 38).

The incidence of PTCL in the USA is less than 1 per 100 000 according to the latest Surveillance, Epidemiology, and End Results (SEER) registry.[1] Here, 'T/natural killer (NK)-cell lymphoid neoplasms' accounted for 6% of all lymphoid neoplasms (B-cell lymphoid neoplasms accounted for 80% and Hodgkin lymphoma for 7%). During 1997–2006, the incidence of T/NK-cell lymphoid neoplasms in the SEER registry was tenfold lower than that of B-cell lymphoid neoplasms (2.09 vs 27.96 per 100 000). The incidence was highest for PTCL (0.78), followed by mycosis fungoides/Sézary syndrome (0.54) and T/NK-cell lymphoid neoplasms not otherwise specified (NOS) (0.49).

While the incidence of lymphoid neoplasms as a whole appears to have plateaued in the USA during 1997–2006, this largely reflects slowing in the rate of increase of B-cell neoplasms, particularly in white men. Rates of T/NK-cell lymphoid neoplasms rose by 1.17% annually, and higher rates were seen in black men (2.2%) and Asian women (2.3%). The rate of PTCL increased by 3.78% over this time, with markedly greater increases in AITL (14%) and PTCL-NOS (5.5%). There was a decrease in the incidence of ALCL (2.0%) but this, and the concomitant increase in AITL, may have been related to changes in coding.

In the UK, approximately 1000 people were diagnosed with PTCL in England and Wales in 2008, representing 10% of approximately 10 000 cases of non-Hodgkin lymphoma.[2]

The incidence of the different subtypes of PTCL in the SEER registry is shown in Table 3.1.

The overall frequency of the different subtypes of PTCL from the International PTCL project are shown in Table 3.2, based on retrospective analysis of 1314 cases of previously untreated PTCL or ENKTCL diagnosed between 1990 and 2002 at 22 centers worldwide.

TABLE 3.1

Incidence of PTCL subtypes in the USA

Subtype	Incidence (cases per 100 000)
PTCL-NOS	0.41
ALCL	0.28
AITL	0.10
ATLL	0.04
HSTCL	0.01
Enteropathy type	0.01

Source: Wang & Vose, 2013.[1]

TABLE 3.2

Incidence of key PTCL subtypes in the International PTCL Project

Subtype		Frequency (%)
PTCL-NOS		25.9
AITL		18.5
ALCL	ALK+	6.6
	ALK−	5.5
ENKTCL		10.4
Enteropathy-associated		4.7
HSTCL		1.4

Source: Vose et al., 2018.[3]

Demographics

PTCL affects twice as many men as women. Diagnosis is most often in the sixth and seventh decades of life, except for HSTCL, which occurs most frequently in younger and middle-aged men receiving immunosuppressive treatment.

Ethnic differences

Based on the 1997–2006 SEER data, rates of nodal PTCL are, generally, highest in black ethnic groups, followed by white and Asian groups, for both men and women (Figure 3.1); however, the pattern varies with subtype. For example, the frequency of AITL is higher among Asian men than black or white men.

A study of 13 107 cases of PTCL in SEER registries between 2000 and 2012 reported that the annual incidence was highest in black people and lowest in Native Americans.[5] Differences in the distribution of the different subtypes were also reported (all $p < 0.05$).

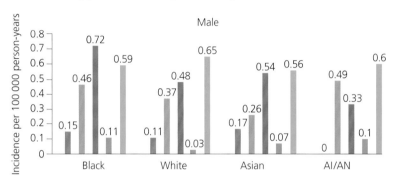

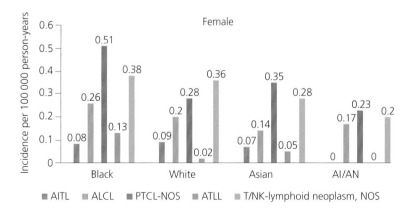

Figure 3.1 Frequency of PTCL by race and sex in the USA, 1997–2006. Values are incidence per 100 000 person-years, adjusted to the 2000 US population. AI/AN, American Indian/Alaskan Native. Based on data from the Surveillance, Epidemiology, and End Results registry.[4]

- The incidence of PTCL-NOS, ALCL and ATLL was higher in black than in non-Hispanic white people, whereas the incidence of AITL was lower.
- Asians/Pacific Islanders had a higher incidence of AITL, ATLL, nasal-type ENKTCL and NK-cell leukemia, and a lower incidence of ALCL.
- Hispanic people had a higher incidence of AITL and ENKTCL.
- Native Americans had a lower incidence of PTCL-NOS.

Survival also varied significantly by race/ethnicity ($p < 0.001$): for most subtypes, survival was generally shorter in black people.

Geographic distribution

The frequency of the most common subtypes of PTCL varies geographically.[3,6]

- In Europe, the nodal subtypes account for more than 80% of PTCL cases in Caucasian patients (PTCL-NOS 34%; AITL 28%; ALK+ ALCL 6%; ALK– ALCL 9%).
- PTCL-NOS is more common in North America but less common in Europe and East Asia.
- AITL is more common in Europe than in Asia or North America.
- For ALCL, the ALK+ form is more common in North America whereas the ALK– form is more common in Europe.
- EATL is more common in areas with a high incidence of celiac disease – it accounts for 5.8% and 9.1% of PTCLs in North America and Europe, respectively, but only 1.9% in Asia. This reflects its close association with the DQ HLA that results in overt or silent celiac disease.
- EBV-associated lymphoproliferative T- and NK-cell neoplasms (e.g. ENKTCL) are more commonly seen in East Asian countries such as Korea and northern China, and in Native American populations from South and Central America.
- The distribution of lymphomas associated with human T-cell lymphotropic virus type 1 (HTLV-1) reflects the distribution of the virus, notably Japan and the Caribbean basin (see below).

Viral infections implicated in T-cell lymphomas

As noted above, the increasing incidence of ENKTCL in East Asia is partly due to endemic HTLV-1 and Epstein–Barr virus (EBV) infections. Although ENKTCL is substantially more common in East Asian and

South American territories, this cannot be explained by differences in EBV seroprevalence – EBV is endemic, infecting 95% of adults globally. The higher incidence may be related to as-yet unidentified genetic factors or environmental cofactors.

HTLV-1. Lymphomas associated with HTLV-1 include ATLL, smoldering ATLL (small numbers of circulating leukemia cells but no nodal involvement), lymphomatous ATLL (lymphadenopathy but no leukemia involvement) and chronic ATLL.

EBV. Demographic and biological data support the early involvement of EBV in the initiation and potentiation of ENKTCL. The virus is present in clonal form in virtually all cases of ENKTCL and aggressive NK leukemia, irrespective of ethnicity.[7] However, genetic and environmental oncogenic cofactors are likely to be involved in the pathogenesis. EBV may also contribute to the transformation of Tfh cells in AITL. EBV has also been detected in most AITL biopsies, although the majority of the EBV-harboring cells are polyclonal B cells; the malignant T cells are EBV-negative.[8] Interestingly, EBV-positive aggressive B-cell lymphomas are well known to arise in the later stages of AITL.[9]

The human herpes virus HHV6B is detectable in half of the cases of AITL, but its role in pathogenesis is unclear. These viruses may modulate expression or function of cytokines, chemokines and membrane receptors in AITL.

Key points – epidemiology and etiology

- T-cell lymphomas are rare, representing approximately 10% of all non-Hodgkin lymphomas.
- PTCL subtypes display marked variation in geographic distribution; AITL and EATL are more frequent in Europe whereas ATLL is more common in Japan and the Caribbean basin and ENKTCL in South East Asia.
- Human T-cell lymphotropic virus type 1 is strongly implicated in lymphomagenesis in ATLL, and Epstein–Barr virus in ENKTCL.

Key references

1. Wang SS, Vose JM. Epidemiology and prognosis of T-cell lymphoma. In: Foss F, ed. *T-Cell Lymphomas. Contemporary Hematology.* New York: Springer, 2013:25–39.

2. NICE. *Pralatrexate for the treatment of relapsed or refractory peripheral T-cell lymphoma.* 2011. www.nice.org.uk/guidance/gid-tag424/documents/lymphoma-non-hodgkins-peripheral-tcell-pralatrexate-draft-scope2, last accessed 15 May 2019.

3. Vose J, Armitage J, Weisenburger D, International TCLP. International peripheral T-cell and natural killer/T-cell lymphoma study: pathology findings and clinical outcomes. *J Clin Oncol* 2008;26:4124–30.

4. Wang L, Wang ZH, Chen XQ et al. First-line combination of gemcitabine, oxaliplatin, and L-asparaginase (GELOX) followed by involved-field radiation therapy for patients with stage IE/IIE extranodal natural killer/T-cell lymphoma. *Cancer* 2013;119:348–55.

5. Adams SV, Newcomb PA, Shustov AR. Racial patterns of peripheral T-cell lymphoma incidence and survival in the United States. *J Clin Oncol* 2016;34:963–71.

6. d'Amore F, Gaulard P, Trumper L et al. Peripheral T-cell lymphomas: ESMO Clinical Practice Guidelines for diagnosis, treatment and follow-up. *Ann Oncol* 2015;26 Suppl 5:v108–15.

7. Au WY, Weisenburger DD, Intragumtornchai T et al. Clinical differences between nasal and extranasal natural killer/T-cell lymphoma: a study of 136 cases from the International Peripheral T-Cell Lymphoma Project. *Blood* 2009;113:3931–7.

8. Weiss LM, Jaffe ES, Liu XF et al. Detection and localization of Epstein-Barr viral genomes in angioimmunoblastic lymphadenopathy and angioimmunoblastic lymphadenopathy-like lymphoma. *Blood* 1992;79:1789–95.

9. Zettl A, Lee SS, Rudiger T et al. Epstein–Barr virus-associated B-cell lymphoproliferative disorders in angiommunoblastic T-cell lymphoma and peripheral T-cell lymphoma, unspecified. *Am J Clin Pathol* 2002;117:368–79.

4 Diagnosis

Accurate diagnosis and subtyping of PTCL is challenging but crucial, because it determines both prognosis and choice of therapy. The neoplastic nature of a given T-cell population is informed by its morphology, aberrant T-cell phenotype and clonality based on T-cell receptor (TCR) genotype[1] (i.e. $\alpha\beta$ versus $\gamma\delta$; see page 11). Accumulating evidence indicates that TCR genotype and the cell of origin influence tumor biology and clinical behavior, and are becoming increasingly clinically relevant as targeted therapeutic options emerge. Distinction between the PTCL subtypes requires consideration of the clinical picture, morphology, immunohistochemistry, flow cytometry, cytogenetics and molecular biology.

Presentation

The symptoms of PTCL vary widely. Often, however, the only sign is an enlarged painless lymph node in the neck, armpit or groin. Some patients also experience generalized (constitutional) symptoms, known as B symptoms, which may include unexplained recurrent fevers over weeks, severe night sweats and significant unexplained weight loss. In the COMPLETE study, 46% of patients presented with B symptoms.[2]

Skin rash may be present, particularly in patients with PTCL-NOS or AITL. Patients with AITL may also present with hypotension, fevers, rash and vasculitis-like symptoms, due to tumor-related cytokine release.

Some patients have more subtle symptoms, such as loss of appetite and fatigue, or symptoms specific to the type of lymphoma, such as joint pains resembling arthritis (which can be migratory), difficulty breathing or persistent dry cough. The liver or spleen may be enlarged. Characteristic presentations of the different subtypes of PTCL are shown in Table 4.1.

TABLE 4.1

Clinical manifestations of PTCL subtypes

Subtype	Typical clinical presentation
AITL and PTCL-NOS	Lymphadenopathy, B symptoms, extranodal involvement, skin rash
ALCL	Lymphadenopathy, extranodal involvement, including bone lesions
ATLL	Lymphadenopathy, hypercalcemia, bone lesions, extranodal involvement
EATL	Abdominal pain, malabsorption, bowel obstruction or perforation
ENKTCL	Nasal stuffiness/discharge, hard palate perforation
HSTCL	Hepatosplenomegaly, pancytopenia, fevers

Examination and diagnostic work-up

Table 4.2 presents an overview of clinical evaluation, based on the MD Anderson Cancer Center practice algorithm[3] and elaborated with the authors' clinical experience. Practice is likely to vary between centers.

During physical examination, particular attention should be paid to lymph node groups, including Waldeyer's ring, and to the size of the liver and spleen. B symptoms should be evaluated and performance status determined. Cardiac evaluation is required prior to chemotherapy.

Biopsy

Lymph node biopsy is essential. Either a core needle biopsy or, preferably, excision of the node is recommended to allow visualization of the broad pattern of lymph node infiltration. Fine needle aspirate is not sufficient for the diagnosis of T-cell lymphomas. Multiple cores should be obtained where possible, given the heterogeneity of many T-cell lymphomas, and to obtain adequate tissue for flow cytometry.

TABLE 4.2

Clinical evaluation in PTCL

Essential	Useful in selected cases
• Physical examination, particularly node-bearing areas and skin	• Brain MRI and lumbar puncture if clinical suspicion and/or high risk of CNS disease
• IPI, performance status, B symptoms	• EBV qPCR on peripheral blood and/or EBER ISH on biopsy if ENKTCL, aggressive NK leukemia or AITL is suspected*
• Complete and differential blood count, platelets, blood urea nitrogen, creatinine, albumin, AST, bilirubin, alkaline phosphatase, serum calcium, uric acid, LDH	• Serum immunoelectrophoresis
	• Direct antiglobulin test where evidence of hemolysis (seen in 15% of cases of AITL)
• Bone marrow biopsy	• CMV IgG if alemtuzumab is considered
• Left ventricular ejection fraction (Muga scan or echocardiogram)	• Pregnancy test
• CT of neck, chest, abdomen and pelvis and/or PET-CT	• Discuss fertility options and sperm banking for patients of child-bearing potential
• Screening for hepatitis B and C (HBcAb, HBaAg, HCVAb)	
• Screening for HIV (when appropriate and according to local guidelines)	
• Screening for HTLV-1 in areas where the virus is endemic (Asia, South America, Caribbean basin) and in areas with diverse demographics	

Based on the MD Anderson Cancer Center practice algorithm[3] and elaborated with the authors' clinical experience. Practice is likely to vary between centers.
*EBV screening is not appropriate because 95% of adults globally are seropositive.
AST, aspartate aminotransferase; CMV IgG, cytomegalovirus immunoglobulin G; CNS, central nervous system; EBER ISH, Epstein–Barr virus encoding region in situ hybridization; EBV, Epstein–Barr virus; HBAb/Ag, hepatitis B antibody/antigen; HCVAb, hepatitis C virus antibody; HIV, human immunodeficiency virus; HTLV-1, human T-cell lymphotropic virus 1; IPI, International Prognostic Index; LDH, lactate dehydrogenase; PET, positron emission tomography; qPCR, quantitative polymerase chain reaction.

The initial immunohistochemistry panel should include: CD20, CD10, CD3, CD30, CD4, CD8, CD7, CD2, CD56, CD21, CD23, BCL6, Ki-67, ALK, TCRB and TCRg. Epstein–Barr virus (EBV) encoding region (EBER) in situ hybridization (ISH) should be considered in cases suspected to be nasal ENKTCL. Molecular analysis should include TCR gene rearrangements, and fluorescence ISH to detect genetic alterations. *DUSP22* and *TP63* rearrangement studies should be considered in patients with ALK⁻ ALCL, as this may affect prognosis.

Bone marrow biopsy. Because 30% of PTCL-NOS cases show bone marrow involvement, a biopsy is recommended as part of initial staging in all patients. Bone marrow aspirate should also be sent for flow cytometry and gene rearrangement studies.

Imaging

Total body imaging is required for accurate staging. Imaging at diagnosis should include cross-sectional imaging of the neck, chest, abdomen and pelvis, conventionally by contrast-enhanced CT, but increasingly using functional fluorodeoxyglucose (FDG) PET-CT. PET-CT is particularly useful for imaging extranodal PTCL and types of T-cell lymphoma presenting in the skin, and is recommended at staging and restaging; however, residual FDG-avid lesions lack specificity, and biopsy confirmation is recommended.

Histopathology

Histopathological analysis by an experienced hematopathologist is key to correct diagnosis and classification. Table 4.3 presents an overview of pathological diagnosis based on the MD Anderson Cancer Center practice algorithm[3] and elaborated with the authors' clinical experience. Practice is likely to vary between centers.

Interpretation. The immunophenotypes of PTCL, TCR rearrangement and putative cell of origin are shown in Table 2.2 (page 19). Specific markers may be relevant to the classification of particular T-cell lymphomas.

- The presence of at least three of the following markers indicates follicular T-helper cell origin: CD10, BCL-6, CXCL13, PD1, SAP, ICOS and CCR5; however, morphology should also be evaluated before diagnosing AITL.

TABLE 4.3

Pathological diagnosis of PTCL

Core	Extended

• Adequate morphology and immunophenotyping to establish diagnosis
  – Paraffin panel: CD20, CD3, CD4, CD8 and other pan-T-cell markers (CD2, CD5, CD7, CD43) and Ki-67
or
  – Flow cytometry immunophenotypic studies: CD2, CD3, CD4, CD5, CD7, CD8, CD10, CD16, CD25, CD26, CD14, CD45, CD52, CD56, CD57, CD94, TCR β and γ
• Molecular studies to detect clonality of TCR genes
	• EBER ISH – NK malignancies and AITL
	• CD16, CD56, CD57 – NK malignancies
	• Cytotoxic proteins (TIA-1, granzyme B, perforin) – NK malignancies and subset of PTCL-NOS
	• BetaF1, TCRγ – $\gamma\delta$ T-cell lymphomas
	• CD10, BCL-6, PD1, CXCL13, ICOS – AITCL
	• CD30, CD15, ALK1, EMA – ALCL
	• CD103 – EATCL
	• CD1a, CD34, TdT – T lymphoblastic lymphoma
	• TCL-1, FoxP3, CD25 – T-cell prolymphocytic leukemia; adult T-cell leukemia/lymphoma

Based on the MD Anderson Cancer Center practice algorithm[3] and elaborated with the authors' clinical experience. Practice is likely to vary between centers.
EBER ISH, Epstein–Barr virus encoding region in situ hybridization; NK, natural killer; TCR, T-cell receptor, Markers are defined in the list of abbreviations (page 4).

- CD21 and/or CD23 are useful in revealing follicular dendritic cells in AITL.
- CD56 is helpful in differentiating between EATL and MEITL (CD8$^+$/CD56$^-$ vs CD8$^-$/CD56$^+$); MEITL typically expresses a $\gamma\delta$-TCR phenotype and is not associated with celiac disease.
- CD30 is always positive in ALCL, which is invariably PAX5$^-$ and often EMA$^+$, and one-third of cases are CD45$^-$. ALCL is further

categorized as ALK+ or ALK- depending on the presence or absence of the t(2;5) translocation (or one of its variants).

- CD30 is variably positive in selected patients with other types of T-cell lymphoma, including EATL, AITL and PTCL-NOS.
- CD20 and PAX5 allow the identification of B-cell components and can help in distinguishing ALK- ALCL from morphologically aggressive classic Hodgkin lymphoma (PAX5+) with anaplastic features.
- CD68 visualizes the histiocytic component, which may outnumber the neoplastic cell population (e.g. lymphoepithelioid PTCL-NOS, Lennert's variant and the lymphohistiocytic variant of ALCL).
- Cytotoxic markers (TIA-1, granzyme B and perforin) are expressed in NK and γδ T-cell lymphomas and may indicate more aggressive clinical behavior.
- EBV may be detected in a subset of patients with PTCL-NOS, AITL and in all cases of ENKTCL.

Diagnostic pitfalls

- TCR clonality alone should be used with caution to establish or refute a diagnosis of PTCL. TCR clonality is negative in 20% of AITL cases, likely to be because of low tumor burden and contamination by non-malignant stromal cells. Conversely, TCR clonality can be positive in reactive entities, including autoimmune conditions and viral infections.
- ALK+ ALCL with small cell morphology (5–10% of cases) can be confused with CD30+ PTCL-NOS if ALK staining is not performed.
- Up to 30% of AITL cases may demonstrate clonal immunoglobulin heavy chain rearrangements but this does not fulfil the criteria for a composite B-cell lymphoma. Composite diffuse large B-cell lymphoma (DLBCL) with AITL should be considered in the presence of sheet-like growth of large monoclonal B cells.
- Hodgkin-like or Reed–Sternberg-like cells in AITL can mimic classic Hodgkin lymphoma. These cells are activated, usually EBV+, B cells.[4]
- Some reactive entities such as infectious mononucleosis, progressive transformation of germinal centers and Kikuchi disease can mimic PTCL.[5]

Staging and grading

Most PTCLs are aggressive, so grading per se may not be relevant. Low-grade T-cell non-Hodgkin lymphoma (NHL) is uncommon and not well described.

The Ann Arbor staging system used to stage lymphomas (Table 4.4) is analogous to the tumor, nodes, metastases (TNM) system used for solid tumors. The clinical stage depends on where malignant tissue is identified and the presence of systemic B symptoms.

TABLE 4.4

Ann Arbor staging system for PTCL

Stage	Involvement	Extranodal status
I/IE	Single node/group of adjacent nodes or lymphoid structure	Single limited extra-lymphatic site
II/IIE	≥2 nodal regions on same side of diaphragm	Stage I or II with limited contiguous extranodal involvement
IIE	As II, with involvement of a contiguous limited extralymphatic site	Not applicable
III	Nodal regions or lymphatic structures on both sides of diaphragm	
IV	Diffuse involvement of ≥1 extralymphatic site ± associated nodal involvement	
Modifiers	E: extranodal involvement (stages I and II only)	
	A/B: absence/presence of systemic B symptoms (see page 41)	
	X: bulky disease (>1/3 widening of mediastinum at T5 or 6, or nodal mass >10 cm; histology and prognostic factors may inform staging	
	S: splenic involvement	

Lymphatic tissues: lymph nodes, Waldeyer's ring, spleen, appendix, thymus, Peyer patches. Nodal tissues: tonsils, Waldeyer's ring, spleen.

Prognostication

PTCL is usually aggressive, and outcomes are generally poor compared with aggressive B-cell lymphomas. For example, the International T-cell Lymphoma study reported overall survival (OS) and failure-free survival of 10% at 10–15 years in patients with PTCL-NOS.[6] Chemokine expression and proliferative signature have been shown to have prognostic significance (Table 4.5).

Several prognostic indices have been developed, informed by studies which identified risk factors that predicted OS and progression-free survival (Table 4.6).

The International Prognostic Index (IPI) was developed in 1993 to identify factors that predict the prognosis of patients with aggressive NHL, as Ann Arbor stage alone did not adequately predict survival outcomes. The IPI has been shown to predict survival in patients with ALCL, AITL and PTCL-NOS, but not for other PTCL entities, and is the most commonly used prognostic index for T-cell lymphoma.

TABLE 4.5

Prognostic significance of biological factors in PTCL

Worse	Favorable	Variable
p53	NF-κB	CXCR3
Ki-67	CCR3	
BCL-2, BCL-XL	ALK-1	
CD26	TCR BF1	
EBV		
MDR		
CCND2		
CCR4		
PRDM1		
TCR δ1		

Definitions of the biological markers are provided in the list of abbreviations (page 4). Adapted from Foss et al. 2011.[7]

TABLE 4.6

Prognostic indices used in PTCL

System	Risk factors	Risk groups (5-year OS)
International Prognostic Index (IPI)	One point for each risk factor: • Age >60 years • Stage III or IV disease • Elevated serum LDH • PS ≥2 • >1 extranodal site	• 0–1 points: low risk (73%) • 2 points: low–intermediate risk (51%) • 3 points: intermediate–high (43%) • 4–5 points: high risk (26%)
Prognostic Index for T-cell Lymphomas (PIT) for PTCL-NOS[8]	• Age > 60 years • Normal or elevated serum LDH • PS ≥2 • Bone marrow involvement	Number of risk factors • 0 (62%) • 1 (53%) • 2 (33%) • >2 (18%)
Modified PIT for PTCL-NOS[9]	• Age >60 years • Normal or elevated serum LDH • PS ≥2 • Ki-67 ≥80%	• Good • Intermediate • Poor
T cell score[10]	• Serum albumin • PS ≥2 • Stage • Absolute neutrophil count	Score: risk (3-year OS) • 0: low (76%) • 1–2: intermediate (43%) • 3–4: high (11%)

LDH, lactate dehydrogenase; OS, overall survival; PS, performance status.

The Prognostic Index for T-cell Lymphomas (PIT) was developed in an attempt to produce more accurate prognostic indicators for PTCL subtypes.[8] Retrospective univariate analysis of data from 385 PTCL-NOS cases identified factors associated with worse OS as:

- age > 60 years
- ≥ 2 extranodal sites
- elevated or normal lactate dehydrogenase (LDH)
- performance status ≥ 2
- stage III or IV disease
- bone marrow involvement.

Multivariate analysis identified four independent risk factors – age, serum LDH, OS and bone marrow involvement. These were used to construct a prognostic model that stratified patients into four groups with 0, 1, 2 or more than 2 risk factors, with 5-year OS rates of 62%, 53%, 33% and 18%, respectively.

The modified Prognostic Index for T-cell Lymphoma (mPIT) replaced bone marrow involvement with expression of the proliferation-associated protein Ki-67. mPIT distinguishes good, intermediate and poor risk groups.[9]

T cell score. The International T cell Project, established by the International Peripheral T-cell Lymphoma Project in 2006, reported this new prognostic model in 2018. It is based on four of 12 explored covariates that maintained their prognostic value in multiple Cox proportional hazards regression analyses: serum albumin, performance status, stage and absolute neutrophil count. Three groups were identified: low risk (score 0; 48 patients [15%]), intermediate risk (score 1–2; 189 patients [61%]) and high risk (score 3–4; 74 patients [24%]), with 3-year OS rates of 76%, 43% and 11%, respectively.[10]

Key points – diagnosis

- Many patients with aggressive T-cell lymphomas present with systemic symptoms, and extranodal involvement is common.
- Detailed immunophenotypic analysis is necessary to accurately diagnose PTCL subtypes.
- PET scanning can be helpful to diagnose extranodal disease.
- The International Prognostic Index and the PTCL-specific index are useful prognostic tools.
- Epstein–Barr virus and CD30 are expressed in several subtypes of PTCL.

Key references

1. Gaulard P, de Leval L. Pathology of peripheral T-cell lymphomas: where do we stand? *Semin Hematol* 2014;51:5–16.

2. Carson KR, Horwitz SM, Pinter-Brown LC et al. A prospective cohort study of patients with peripheral T-cell lymphoma in the United States. *Cancer* 2017;123:1174–83.

3. MD Anderson Cancer Center. *Peripheral T-cell lymphomas (PTCL) practice algorithm.* 2017. www.mdanderson.org/documents/for-physicians/algorithms/cancer-treatment/ca-treatment-lymphoma-peripheral-t-cell-web-algorithm.pdf, last accessed 15 May 2019.

4. Nicolae A, Pittaluga S, Venkataraman G et al. Peripheral T-cell lymphomas of follicular T-helper cell derivation with Hodgkin/Reed-Sternberg cells of B-cell lineage: both EBV-positive and EBV-negative variants exist. *Am J Surg Pathol* 2013;37:816–26.

5. Zhang XY, Collins GP, Soilleux E, Eyre TA. Acute EBV masquerading as peripheral T-cell lymphoma. *BMJ Case Rep* 2016;2016.

6. Vose J, Armitage J, Weisenburger D, International TCLP. International peripheral T-cell and natural killer/T-cell lymphoma study: pathology findings and clinical outcomes. *J Clin Oncol* 2008;26:4124–30.

7. Foss FM, Zinzani PL, Vose JM et al. Peripheral T-cell lymphoma. *Blood* 2011;117:6756–67.

8. Gallamini A, Stelitano C, Calvi R et al. Peripheral T-cell lymphoma unspecified (PTCL-U): a new prognostic model from a retrospective multicentric clinical study. *Blood* 2004;103:2474–9.

9. Went P, Agostinelli C, Gallamini A et al. Marker expression in peripheral T-cell lymphoma: a proposed clinical-pathologic prognostic score. *J Clin Oncol* 2006;24:2472–9.

10. Federico M, Bellei M, Marcheselli L et al. Peripheral T cell lymphoma, not otherwise specified (PTCL-NOS). A new prognostic model developed by the International T cell Project Network. *Br J Haematol* 2018;181:760–69.

5 First-line treatment

PTCL is invariably fatal within a few months without treatment. Wherever possible, treatment aims to achieve long-term cure using chemotherapy and, in some situations, hemopoietic stem cell transplantation (see Chapter 7). First-line treatment offers the most realistic chance of achieving cure. Relapsed and refractory PTCL is associated with dire clinical outcomes.

Conventional chemotherapy regimens showing activity in aggressive lymphomas (predominantly B-cell lymphomas) in the 1990s evolved to become the de facto standard of care for PTCL. Progress in developing specific treatments for PTCL has been hampered by the rarity of the diseases, the substantial clinical and biological heterogeneity of the subtypes, compounded by insufficient understanding of the molecular pathobiology, and a lack of the definitive clinical trial data from comparative studies that is needed to change practice. There is no standard 'one size fits all' treatment – the therapeutic approach varies across and within individual countries and for defined disease entities.

At present, the nodal PTCLs (PTCL-NOS, AITL, follicular helper T cell [Tfh]-related lymphomas, ALK⁻ ALCL), which account for most PTCL cases, are treated using the uniform approaches outlined below. PTCL subtypes that require distinct treatment strategies are discussed separately (pages 56–9).

Importantly, individual PTCL cases require expert hematopathology review to ensure accurate subtyping (see Chapter 4), together with input from a multidisciplinary lymphoma team with experience in the diagnosis and management of PTCL. Prognostic score, performance status and relevant comorbidities should be considered for each patient before deciding on treatment. Given that clinical outcomes are generally poor, involvement in a therapeutic clinical study should be considered whenever possible. Patients should also be offered the opportunity to contribute to regional or national PTCL biobanks, an essential resource for translational studies.

First-line treatment for nodal PTCL

CHOP chemotherapy (Table 5.1) became the backbone of treatment for aggressive non-Hodgkin lymphoma on the basis of large Phase III trials that confirmed activity and survival benefit compared with historic regimens. However, these trials mostly included patients with aggressive B-cell malignancies, and the superiority of CHOP over alternative chemotherapy regimens in PTCL has never been demonstrated prospectively. In fact, retrospective analysis of cases from the international T-cell Lymphoma Project did not show any survival benefit with anthracycline-based chemotherapy in patients with PTCL.[1] Outcomes with CHOP are unsatisfactory for patients with PTCL: whilst initial complete responses are seen in 40–70% of patients, most develop refractory or relapsed disease, typically within 1–2 years of diagnosis.

Intensified regimens have been used in an attempt to overcome the poor outcomes seen with CHOP. Whilst some Phase II trials have shown good outcomes with intensified protocols, these have not been randomized studies against CHOP, making it difficult to draw conclusions. The only randomized Phase III trial comparing CHOP with an intensive regimen of VIP combined with the ABVD backbone in 88 patients did not show any improvement in survival (5-year event-free survival [EFS]: 32.5% vs 32%).[2]

TABLE 5.1

CHOP chemotherapy

Agent	Route	Dose	Dosing in 21-day cycle*
Cyclophosphamide	Intravenous	750 mg/m²	1
Hydroxydaunorubicin (doxorubicin)	Intravenous	50 mg/m²	1
Vincristine	Intravenous	1.4 mg/m² to a maximum of 2 mg	1
Prednisolone	Oral	100 mg	1–5

*Although CHOP is typically administered on a 21-day cycle, some centers advocate a 14-day cycle to achieve dose density. Typically, six cycles are administered.

Modifying CHOP. Rather than replacing CHOP, further chemotherapy or non-chemotherapy agents have been added to the CHOP backbone, or have replaced agents in CHOP, in attempts to improve clinical outcomes.

CHOEP. Retrospective analysis of patients with PTCL treated with several high-grade lymphoma trial protocols found that, in younger patients (< 60 years) with normal lactate dehydrogenase (LDH) levels, the addition of etoposide, 100 mg/m² intravenously on days 1–3, to CHOP (CHOEP) significantly improved EFS (75.4% vs 51%; $p = 0.003$).[3] However, 60% of these patients had ALCL, and a post-hoc subgroup analysis showed that this benefit held only for younger patients with ALK⁺ ALCL.

Swedish population data also demonstrated a progression-free survival (PFS) advantage with CHOEP in younger patients.[4] No study has found an overall survival (OS) benefit, and the addition of etoposide to CHOP increases toxicity. Despite these caveats, CHOEP has been widely adopted as a standard first-line treatment for PTCL.

MegaCHOEP (high-dose CHOP and etoposide) did not prevent early progression in a small cohort of younger, fit patients with PTCL treated in German clinical trials, with a complete response rate similar to that reported with standard CHOP, and a 3-year EFS of only 26%.[5]

CHOP + alemtuzumab. Alemtuzumab is a humanized monoclonal antibody to CD52, which is expressed by most AITL and PTCL-NOS cases and half of ALCL cases. High response rates with alemtuzumab–CHOP were reported in Phase II/III studies, whereas EFS was comparable to reported outcomes with CHOP alone but with significantly increased toxicity.[6]

Brentuximab vedotin is a CD30-specific monoclonal antibody conjugated with the toxin monomethyl auristatin E (see pages 69–70), which is administered in combination with CHP chemotherapy (known as CHP+A).[7] A large randomized Phase III trial (ECHELON-2) in patients with CD30⁺ PTCL (≥10%, as assessed by local centers) recently evaluated the benefit of replacing the vincristine in CHOP with brentuximab vedotin, 1.8 mg/kg intravenously on day 1 of each 15-day cycle. The study met the primary endpoint, with CHP + A conferring a significantly improved PFS at 3 years compared with CHOP (57% vs 44%; $p = 0.011$) and a 34% decrease in all-cause mortality. In line with other studies of brentuximab vedotin, a correlation was not found between response and level of CD30 expression. Seventy percent of the trial participants had systemic ALCL, which does not reflect typical clinical practice but was a regulatory condition for the trial.

CHP+A is likely to become a new standard of care as first-line therapy for this PTCL subgroup but the study was not powered to detect differences in outcome in non-ALCL subtypes. Nevertheless, the Food and Drug Administration approved CHP+A in November 2018 for previously untreated systemic ALCL and CD30-expressing PTCL; a decision from the European Medicines Agency was pending at the time of publication.

Alternative chemotherapy backbones. The underlying mechanisms that mediate CHOP chemoresistance in PTCL are not well understood but one possible explanation is the high expression of P glycoprotein pumps (PGP; *MDR1* gene). Cell surface expression of these drug efflux pumps may rapidly transport anthracyclines and vinca alkaloids out of the lymphoma cell, causing resistance. Chemotherapeutic agents that bypass this resistance mechanism have therefore been explored as alternative first-line strategies.

Gemcitabine is a nucleoside analog that is not a substrate for PGP and has activity in relapsed and refractory PTCL. However, GEM-P was not superior to CHOP in a recent UK randomized Phase II trial,[8] and PEGS achieved 2-year PFS of only 12% in a Phase II trial (80% of patients with newly diagnosed PTCL).[9]

Treatment of limited-stage PTCL

Very few patients present with limited-stage nodal PTCL, and there is a paucity of data guiding clinical management. Data suggest that, with the exception of ALK+ ALCL, limited-stage PTCL is associated with worse outcomes than limited-stage diffuse large B-cell lymphoma (DLBCL).

Treatment options include standard induction chemotherapy as described above, or a short course of CHOP-like chemotherapy (3 or 4 cycles) with involved-site radiotherapy. The decision to reduce chemotherapy and use radiotherapy requires careful consideration of toxicity and risks. Radiotherapy alone is highly unlikely to provide adequate treatment for most cases.

Treatment of specific subtypes

ALK⁺ ALCL. Outcomes with CHOP chemotherapy are significantly better in ALK⁺ ALCL than in other PTCL subtypes and are akin to those seen in DLBCL. Younger patients may benefit from the addition of etoposide (see above), whereas in older patients (>60 years) this benefit appears to be offset by greater toxicity. Intensified strategies and consolidation autologous stem cell transplantation are generally reserved for relapsed/refractory disease given potentially favorable clinical outcomes with CHOP-based chemotherapy.

Young age is a major influence on the favorable prognosis of ALK⁺ ALCL. A few patients with ALK⁺ ALCL who present at an older age with other adverse risk factors (e.g. high LDH, extranodal sites) may have poor outcomes, similar to those with ALK⁻ ALCL.

As described above, recent data demonstrating benefit with CHP+A is likely to define a new standard of care for ALCL. Patients with ALK⁺ ALCL were eligible for the pivotal trial only if they had adverse risk factors resulting in an International Prognostic Index score above 2, but showed the greatest benefit with CHP+A compared with other subtypes.

Breast implant-associated ALCL that presents with seroma only, with no evidence of tissue involvement, can often be managed expectantly by careful observation after capsule removal. Where there is evidence of tissue involvement beyond the capsule, patients are generally treated with protocols used for ALK⁻ ALCL. Involvement is bilateral in about 5% of cases, providing a basis for removal of the contralateral implant. Implant replacement should be avoided wherever possible. A few patients have been treated with radiotherapy to the involved field. The roles of brentuximab vedotin and chemotherapy in breast implant-associated ALCL have not been clearly defined.[10]

All cases should be reported to the appropriate regulatory agencies and, where possible, included in national or international registries to support surveillance.

Aggressive intestinal lymphomas. EATL and MEITL are both highly aggressive, with very low response rates to CHOP-like chemotherapy – fewer than 10% of patients achieve long-term survival (i.e. 5 years). An intensified strategy has been developed for EATL, involving an

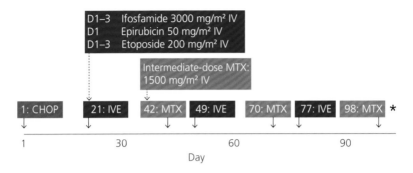

Figure 5.1 Consolidated chemotherapy protocol for the treatment of enteropathy-associated T-cell lymphoma. CHOP is explained in Table 5.1 (page 53). *Autologous stem cell transplantation (ASCT) is performed 4–6 weeks after the last course of IVE/MTX, with high-dose conditioning therapy (BEAM) comprising carmustine, 300 mg/m² on day 1, etoposide, 200 mg/m² on days 2–5, cytarabine (Ara-C), 200 mg/m² twice daily on days 2–5, and melphalan, 140 mg/m² on day 6. IV, intravenously; MTX, methotrexate.

initial cycle of CHOP, followed by alternating IVE and intermediate-dose intravenous methotrexate (Figure 5.1) and consolidation with high-dose therapy (BEAM) and autologous stem cell transplantation.[11] Clinical outcomes were improved compared with historic controls treated with CHOP-like treatment, and this regimen has been adopted by many centers internationally.

HSTCL is extremely rare and highly aggressive, with limited evidence to guide treatment decisions. Most case series consistently report high failure rates with CHOP-like chemotherapy. More intensive regimens, especially those containing etoposide, are typically used, although median survival is typically less than 12 months.[12] Most experts recommend that patients with chemotherapy-sensitive disease should proceed rapidly to consolidative allogeneic stem cell transplantation before disease relapse occurs.

ATLL. Aggressive ATLL is associated with poor clinical outcomes. Patients with newly diagnosed disease are often acutely ill, with poor performance status and high tumor burden. Conventional chemotherapy alone is associated with high failure rates. CHOP-14

(CHOP given every 14 days) achieves initial response in 60–70% of cases but relapse is inevitable and median survival is typically less than a year. Autologous stem cell transplantation does not appear to provide any benefit. Response rates and survival are improved with upfront use of the antiretroviral drug zidovudine and interferon-α, although the greatest benefit is seen in those with acute leukemic disease.[13] These antiviral drugs have a minimal toxicity profile and can be safely combined with chemotherapy regimens. Expert opinion supports early allogeneic stem cell transplantation for eligible patients, given that there are few long-term survivors with chemotherapy alone.

Mogamulizumab is a monoclonal antibody directed against CCR4 (also designated CD194) and has demonstrated significant activity in ATLL (see page 70). In a Japanese study of patients with relapsed/refractory disease, the response rate with mogamulizumab was 50%, with median OS of 13.7 months.[14] A subsequent US randomized study comparing mogamulizumab versus investigator's choice reported overall response rates (ORR) of 28% and 8%, respectively.[15]

A recent study in Japan reported an ORR of 42% with lenalidomide in patients with relapsed or refractory ATLL, with an OS of 20 months.[16]

Patients with aggressive ATLL should be considered for clinical trials where possible.

ENKTCL

Localized disease. Radiotherapy alone achieves an excellent initial response rate, but relapse rates are unacceptably high, suggesting that many patients have occult dissemination. CHOP-based chemotherapy is associated with poor outcomes and should be avoided in patients with ENKTCL. Concurrent or sequential chemoradiotherapy with non-anthracycline-based chemotherapy regimens has demonstrated significant improvements in outcomes. Regimens such as DeVIC (see Table 5.2) with concurrent radiotherapy,[17] GELOX with radiotherapy sandwiched in the middle of chemotherapy[18] and SMILE[19] have achieved complete response rates of 60–80% and 2-year PFS rates above 80%. High radiotherapy doses are required for ENKTCL, typically > 50 Gy.

Advanced disease. The mainstay of treatment is intensive combination chemotherapy that includes asparaginase – an enzyme which breaks down the circulating asparagine that lymphoma cells

TABLE 5.2

Chemotherapy regimens for NK cell malignancies

Regimen	Agent	Dose	Day of cycle
SMILE	Methotrexate	2000 mg/m²	1
	Ifosfamide	1500 mg/m²	
	Dexamethasone	40 mg	2–4
	Etoposide	100 mg/m²	
	L-Asparginase	6000 U/m²	8, 10, 12, 14, 16, 18, 20
DeVIC	Carboplatin	200 mg/m²	1
	Etoposide	67 mg/m²	
	Ifosfamide	1000 mg/m²	1–3
	Dexamathasone	40 mg	

All chemotherapy agents are administered intravenously; dexamethasone may be administered orally in SMILE.
Up to six cycles are administered depending on response, tolerability and plans for consolidative stem cell transplantation.

may depend on. The two most commonly used protocols are SMILE (see Table 5.2) and AspaMetDex.[20] Durable remission is achieved in about half of patients (with or without consolidative stem cell transplantation) but it should be noted that SMILE is an intensive regimen with a treatment-related mortality of 7–10%.

Aggressive NK cell leukemia. Intensive asparaginase-containing protocols such as SMILE are typically used but clinical outcomes are dire, with few long-term survivors. Allogeneic stem cell transplantation should be considered, where feasible, in patients who respond to induction chemotherapy

Radiotherapy

Radiotherapy is typically used as a consolidation strategy following a response to chemotherapy but may be used palliatively if chemotherapy fails. A range of radiotherapy techniques and doses have been used in the management of PTCL depending on tumor location and volume, intent of treatment, and patient characteristics. However, such approaches have largely been adopted empirically from B-cell lymphomas and, with the exception of ENKTCL, very few data are available specifically for PTCL.

Historically, involved-field radiotherapy was used, which encompasses anatomic boundaries including whole lymphatic regions. This is increasingly being replaced by involved-site radiotherapy, which targets a smaller tissue volume encompassing prechemotherapy sites involving lymphoma, with the intention of reducing toxicity. Consolidative radiotherapy to sites of bulk (> 7.5 cm) remains conventional practice. The role of PET-CT imaging to identify patients where radiotherapy can be safely omitted is as yet unclear.

CNS prophylaxis

Data to support clear recommendations for central nervous system (CNS) prophylaxis in patients with PTCL are lacking. Most centers apply the criteria used for aggressive B-cell malignancies, including LDH level, number of extranodal sites, and involvement of specific sites such as testis, kidney or adrenal gland. A CNS International Prognostic Index developed for DLBCL might reasonably be extrapolated to patients with PTCL, although this has not been validated.

Response assessment

The limitations of diagnostic biomarkers in robustly predicting outcomes have driven the search for dynamic response markers. Whilst interim CT scans poorly predict treatment outcomes in lymphoma, functional imaging using PET-CT has garnered much interest. In Hodgkin lymphoma, for example, the use of interim PET (iPET) has changed practice, allowing treatment to be stratified based on the iPET response. iPET has been reported to strongly predict PFS and OS in patients treated with CHOP-like chemotherapy, although these studies were retrospective and included relatively few patients. The prospective PETAL study assessed the clinical utility of iPET before cycle 3 of CHOP in 76 patients with PTCL: 25% were iPET positive and had significantly worse clinical outcomes; intensifying chemotherapy in these patients had no survival benefit.[21]

The integration of iPET with the clearance of circulating tumor DNA has been proposed as a novel composite to better predict outcomes in DLBCL and classic Hodgkin lymphoma.

Key points – first-line treatment

- Insufficient understanding of the pathology of this heterogeneous group of rare diseases, together with a lack of randomized clinical trial data, has hindered progress in the treatment of PTCL, resulting in wide variation in practice.
- The use of intensive treatment strategies for nodal PTCL does not appear to improve outcomes.
- Improved survival with brentuximab vedotin in combination with CHP chemotherapy in the ECHELON-2 trial heralded a new treatment standard in ALCL; however, the benefit in other PTCL subtypes is unclear.
- Extranodal PTCL has a dismal outcome with CHOP-based chemotherapy; alternative therapeutic chemotherapy strategies focused on distinct subtypes are therefore required.

Key references

1. Vose J, Armitage J, Weisenburger D, International TCLP. International peripheral T-cell and natural killer/T-cell lymphoma study: pathology findings and clinical outcomes. *J Clin Oncol* 2008;26: 4124–30.

2. Simon A, Peoch M, Casassus P et al. Upfront VIP-reinforced-ABVD (VIP-rABVD) is not superior to CHOP/21 in newly diagnosed peripheral T cell lymphoma. Results of the randomized phase III trial GOELAMS-LTP95. *Br J Haematol* 2010;151:159–66.

3. Schmitz N, Trumper L, Ziepert M et al. Treatment and prognosis of mature T-cell and NK-cell lymphoma: an analysis of patients with T-cell lymphoma treated in studies of the German High-Grade Non-Hodgkin Lymphoma Study Group. *Blood* 2010;116:3418–25.

4. Ellin F, Landstrom J, Jerkeman M, Relander T. Real-world data on prognostic factors and treatment in peripheral T-cell lymphomas: a study from the Swedish Lymphoma Registry. *Blood* 2014;124:1570–7.

5. Nickelsen M, Ziepert M, Zeynalova S et al. High-dose CHOP plus etoposide (MegaCHOEP) in T-cell lymphoma: a comparative analysis of patients treated within trials of the German High-Grade Non-Hodgkin Lymphoma Study Group (DSHNHL). *Ann Oncol* 2009;20:1977–84.

6. Phillips EH, Devereux S, Radford J et al. Toxicity and efficacy of alemtuzumab combined with CHOP for aggressive T-cell lymphoma: a phase 1 dose-escalation trial. *Leuk Lymph* 2019:1–4.

7. Horwitz S, O'Connor OA, Pro B et al. Brentuximab vedotin with chemotherapy for CD30-positive peripheral T-cell lymphoma (ECHELON-2): a global, double-blind, randomised, phase 3 trial. *Lancet* 2019;393:229–40.

8. Gleeson M, Peckitt C, To YM et al. CHOP versus GEM-P in previously untreated patients with peripheral T-cell lymphoma (CHEMO-T): a phase 2, multicentre, randomised, open-label trial. *Lancet Haematol* 2018;5:e190–200.

9. Mahadevan D, Unger JM, Spier CM et al. Phase 2 trial of combined cisplatin, etoposide, gemcitabine, and methylprednisolone (PEGS) in peripheral T-cell non-Hodgkin lymphoma: Southwest Oncology Group Study S0350. *Cancer* 2013;119:371–9.

10. Mehta-Shah N, Clemens MW, Horwitz SM. How I treat breast implant-associated anaplastic large cell lymphoma. *Blood* 2018;132:1889–98.

11. Sieniawski M, Angamuthu N, Boyd K et al. Evaluation of enteropathy-associated T-cell lymphoma comparing standard therapies with a novel regimen including autologous stem cell transplantation. *Blood* 2010;115:3664–70.

12. Belhadj K, Reyes F, Farcet JP et al. Hepatosplenic γδ T-cell lymphoma is a rare clinicopathologic entity with poor outcome: report on a series of 21 patients. *Blood* 2003;102:4261–9.

13. Hodson A, Crichton S, Montoto S et al. Use of zidovudine and interferon alfa with chemotherapy improves survival in both acute and lymphoma subtypes of adult T-cell leukemia/lymphoma. *J Clin Oncol* 2011;29:4696–701.

14. Ishida T, Joh T, Uike N et al. Defucosylated anti-CCR4 monoclonal antibody (KW-0761) for relapsed adult T-cell leukemia-lymphoma: a multicenter phase II study. *J Clin Oncol* 2012;30:837–42.

15. Phillips AA, Fields PA, Hermine O et al. Mogamulizumab versus investigator's choice of chemotherapy regimen in relapsed/refractory adult T-cell leukemia/lymphoma. *Haematologica* 2019;104:993–1003.

16. Ishida T, Fujiwara H, Nosaka K et al. Multicenter phase II study of lenalidomide in relapsed or recurrent adult T-cell leukemia/lymphoma: ATLL-002. *J Clin Oncol* 2016;34:4086–93.

17. Yamaguchi M, Tobinai K, Oguchi M et al. Phase I/II study of concurrent chemoradiotherapy for localized nasal natural killer/T-cell lymphoma: Japan Clinical Oncology Group Study JCOG0211. *J Clin Oncol* 2009;27:5594–600.

18. Wang L, Wang ZH, Chen XQ et al. First-line combination of gemcitabine, oxaliplatin, and L-asparaginase (GELOX) followed by involved-field radiation therapy for patients with stage IE/IIE extranodal natural killer/T-cell lymphoma. *Cancer* 2013;119:348–55.

19. Kwong YL, Kim WS, Lim ST et al. SMILE for natural killer/T-cell lymphoma: analysis of safety and efficacy from the Asia Lymphoma Study Group. *Blood* 2012;120: 2973–80.

20. Jaccard A, Gachard N, Marin B et al. Efficacy of L-asparaginase with methotrexate and dexamethasone (AspaMetDex regimen) in patients with refractory or relapsing extranodal NK/T-cell lymphoma, a phase 2 study. *Blood* 2011;117:1834–9.

21. Hüttmann A, Müller SP, Rekowski J et al. Positron emission tomography (PET) guided therapy of aggressive lymphomas – interim PET-based outcome prediction and treatment changes in patients with T cell lymphomas participating in the PETAL trial. *Blood* 2016;128:185.

6 Treatment of relapsed and refractory PTCL

Relapsed and refractory PTCL are associated with dismal outcomes, with median overall survival (OS) of 5.3 months reported in a population-based retrospective series of 163 patients from British Columbia.[1] A recent prospective international registry study (the T Cell Project) reported survival outcomes from 633 patients with relapsed or refractory disease following frontline therapy: median OS was 11 months for those with relapsed disease and 5 months for those with refractory disease.[2] Only 16% of this large cohort proceeded to stem cell transplantation. Given these outcomes, treatment within a clinical trial is recommended for patients with relapsed or refractory PTCL.

Several novel agents have recently been approved for the treatment of relapsed and refractory PTCL, and studies are defining how these agents are best used (i.e. as monotherapy or in combination) to improve survival outcomes.

Treatment options

Decisions on the treatment of relapsed or refractory PTCL should first consider whether a patient is a candidate for potentially curative allogeneic stem cell transplantation (see Chapter 7). For these patients the National Comprehensive Cancer Network guidelines recommend either multi- or single-agent chemotherapy for salvage. Patients who are not candidates for transplant should receive single-agent therapy to provide palliative benefit with minimal toxicity.

Multi-agent chemotherapy regimens for PTCL include conventional lymphoma salvage regimens such as ICE, DHAP and ESHAP (Table 6.1). Gemcitabine-based regimens have also shown activity, including GDP, GVD and GemOx.

Single agents

Single agents approved for relapsed or refractory PTCL include pralatrexate,[3] romidepsin[4] and belinostat.[5] Chidamide is a

TABLE 6.1

National Comprehensive Cancer Network guidelines for treatment of relapsed and refractory PTCL

	Single agents (approved)	Other single agents	Combination therapies
Nodal PTCL-NOS, EATL, Tfh-related lymphomas	Belinostat Brentuximab vedotin for CD30+ Pralatrexate Romdepsin	Alemtuzumab Bendamustine Gemcitabine Lenalidomide	DHAP ESHAP GDP GemOx ICE GVD
AITL	Belinostat Brentuximab vedotin for CD30+ Romidepsin	Alemtuzumab Bendamustine Gemcitabine Lenalidomide Pralatrexate	DHAP ESHAP GDP GemOx ICE
ALCL	Belinostat Bendamustine Bortezomib Brentuximab vedotin Gemcitabine Pralatrexate Romidepsin		DHAP ESHAP GDP GemOx ICE GVD

Chemotherapy regimens are defined in the list of abbreviations (page 4).

histone deacetylase (HDAC) inhibitor only approved in China[6] and mogamulizumab is approved for human T-cell lymphotropic virus 1 (HTLV-1)-associated ATLL in Japan.[7] Response rates seen with these treatments are presented in Table 6.2 and their administration and adverse effects in Table 6.3.

Pralatrexate was the first drug for PTCL to be approved by the US Food and Drug Administration (FDA), in 2009.[3] It is a folate analog

TABLE 6.2

Overall response rates (%) with FDA-approved agents

	PTCL-NOS	ALCL	AITL
Prelatrexate (PROPEL)	31	29 Median PFS 3.5 months	8
Romidepsin	29	24	30
Belinostat	23	15 Median PFS 7.9 months	46
Bendamustine	41 Median PFS 3.6 months	50 Median PFS 3.5 months	69
Lenalidomide	33	40 Median PFS 4.0 months	29
Brentuximab vedotin	25 Median PFS 2.6 months	85	50
Alisertib	31	24 Median PFS 3.0 months	Not reported

FDA, Food and Drug Administration; PFS, progression-free survival.

that binds with high affinity to reduced folate carrier-1 and inhibits dihydrofolate reductase, leading to depletion of thymidine monophosphate and other nucleotides, and ultimately inducing apoptosis.

Efficacy. PROPEL was a Phase II single-arm trial of pralatrexate in 115 patients with relapsed or refractory PTCL. Of 111 evaluable patients, 53% had PTCL-NOS, 15% had ALCL and 12% had AITL. Pralatrexate was administered intravenously over 3–5 minutes at 30 mg/m^2 once weekly for 6 weeks, followed by 1 week of rest, until progressive disease or unacceptable toxicity. All patients also received vitamin B12 injections every 2 months and folic acid daily.

TABLE 6.3

Administration and adverse effects of treatments approved for PTCL

Drug	Dose	Tips for administration and AEs
Pralatrexate	30 mg/m² IV weekly for 6 of every 7 weeks	Leucovorin administered day after infusion; daily vitamin B12 and folate required
		Renally excreted; monitor creatinine
		AEs: mucositis, diarrhea, skin rash/ulceration, thrombocytopenia
		Hold or modify dose for grade ≥ 2 mucositis or new skin ulcer
Romidepsin	14 mg/m² IV weekly for 3 of every 4 weeks	ECG pre- and post-dose in first cycle for QTc prolongation
		Avoid other QTc-prolonging agents
		Check potassium and magnesium levels and replete if required
		Administer antinausea medication
		AEs: nausea, fatigue, GI upset, dysgeusia, thrombocytopenia, neutropenia, infections
Belinostat	1000 mg/m² daily for 5 days of 21-day cycle	AEs: nausea, fatigue, GI upset, hematologic toxicity
Brentuximab vedotin	1.8 mg/kg IV every 3 weeks	AEs: peripheral neuropathy, bone marrow suppression, infections, tumor lysis syndrome
		PML from JC virus reported
Mogamulizumab	1 mg/kg weekly for 4 weeks then every 2 weeks	AEs: infusion reactions, skin rash, fatigue, diarrhea
		Rarely, immune-mediated colitis or pneumonitis
		Consider prophylaxis with aciclovir (acyclovir) and bactrim

AE, adverse event; ECG, electrocardiogram; GI, gastrointestinal; IV, intravenous; JCV, John Cunningham virus (a polyomavirus); PML, progressive multifocal leukoencephalopathy.

The overall response rate (ORR) was 29%, including 11% of patients with complete response (CR) and 18% with partial response (PR). Response rates were lower in patients with AITL than in those with PTCL-NOS or ALCL: 8%, 32% and 35%, respectively. The median progression-free survival (PFS) was 3.5 months, and median OS was 14.5 months.

Adverse events. The most frequent adverse events were mucositis, which required dose reductions in 23% of patients and caused withdrawal from treatment in 6%, and cytopenias. Subsequent experience has shown that addition of leucovorin, 25–50 mg, on the day after pralatrexate reduced the incidence of mucositis, and a prospective study of pralatrexate with leucovorin is ongoing.[8]

Histone deacetylase inhibitors were the second class of drugs to be approved for relapsed and refractory PTCL: romidepsin was approved by the FDA in 2011 and belinostat in 2014. Romidepsin is also approved in the USA for the treatment of cutaneous T-cell lymphoma (CTCL). Neither HDAC inhibitor is currently approved in Europe for the treatment of PTCL.

Inhibition of HDAC prevents the acetylation of histone lysine residues, thereby modulating genes responsible for multiple cellular processes, including growth inhibition, cell cycle regulation, apoptosis and immune modulatory pathways. HDAC inhibitors may also alter the post-translational acetylation of proteins in the cytosol, although the exact mechanism of action in T-cell lymphoma is still to be fully elucidated.

Romidepsin is a cyclic tetrapeptide or depsipeptide that inhibits class 1 HDAC. It is approved at a dose of 14 mg/m^2 infused over 4 hours on days 1, 8 and 15 every 28 days, on the basis of two clinical trials.[4,9]

An early trial involving 47 patients with relapsed PTCL reported an ORR of 38% (18% CR) and a median duration of response (DOR) of 8.9 months. A subsequent multicenter single-arm registration study of 130 patients with relapsed or refractory PTCL (including 69 with PTCL-NOS, 27 with AITL and 21 with ALK⁻ ALCL) reported an ORR of 25% (19% CR); the ORR was 29% in PTCL-NOS, 30% in AITL and 24% in ALK⁻ ALCL. Notably, 29% of patients in this study responded to romidepsin despite being refractory to their most recent systemic therapy.[10] Histology, type of prior therapy and prior transplant did not predict response. While the median PFS for the whole cohort was 4 months, it was 18 months in patients who achieved a CR, and CR was sustained for longer than 3 years in some patients.

The most common adverse events included nausea, asthenia and fatigue, thrombocytopenia, infections and diarrhea. Grade 3 or worse events included thrombocytopenia in 24%, neutropenia in 20% and infections in 19%. Electrocardiographic changes (mainly QTc interval prolongation) have been described with romidepsin and other HDAC inhibitors, so care should be taken to exclude other medications that have this effect.

Belinostat is a hydroxamic acid-derived pan-HDAC inhibitor. It is administered at 1000 mg/m², by a short intravenous infusion on days 1–5 of every 21-day cycle. A Phase II study in 24 patients with relapsed or refractory PTCL or CTCL demonstrated an ORR of 25%, with 8% CR.[11] The pivotal single-arm Phase II trial of belinostat in relapsed and refractory PTCL (BELIEF) enrolled 129 patients and reported a similar ORR of 26%, with 11% CR.[5] Notably, the response rate was higher in patients with AITL than in those with ALK⁻ ALCL or PTCL-NOS (ORR 46%, 5% and 23%, respectively). No responses were seen in patients with EATL or HSTCL. For the whole cohort, median PFS and OS were 1.6 months and 7.9 months, respectively. However, responding patients experienced a median DOR of 13.6 months. Twelve patients went on to receive stem cell transplantation.

Adverse events occurring in over 25% of patients were nausea, fatigue, anorexia, anemia and vomiting. Only 12–14% of patients had grade 3 or worse hematologic toxicity, and grade 3 or worse constitutional toxicities (fatigue, asthenia, nausea) occurred in fewer than 3% of patients.

Monoclonal antibodies and immunoconjugates

Brentuximab vedotin is an immunoconjugate comprising a humanized CD30-specific antibody and the microtubule disrupting agent methylauristatin E (MMAE). It binds to the CD30 receptor and is internalized, where it liberates the MMAE fragment into the cytosol to disrupt the microtubule network and induce apoptosis. CD30 is expressed to a varying degree in PTCL, including in about 50% of PTCL-NOS cases, 20% of AITL, and most cases of EATL and ALCL

(ALK⁻ and ALK⁺).[12] It is also thought that small amounts of MMAE are released by tumor cells and affect the tumor microenvironment, potentially explaining the activity of brentuximab vedotin in malignancies with low levels of CD30 expression.

Efficacy and dosage. Brentuximab vedotin is approved in the USA for use in combination with chemotherapy (CHP+A) for previously untreated CD30-expressing subtypes of PTCL, irrespective of the degree of expression of CD30.[13] In Europe, it is approved only for relapsed and refractory systemic ALCL. The standard dose is 1.8 mg/kg every 3 weeks.

A Phase II registration study of brentuximab vedotin as monotherapy in 58 patients with relapsed/refractory ALCL reported an ORR of 86%, with CR in 57% of patients.[14] Median PFS was 13.3 months, and median OS was not reached but was estimated at 64% at 4 years. By design, 70% of participants in the pivotal trial (ECHELON-2) had ALCL so the study was underpowered to identify any significant differences in outcomes in other PTCL subtypes.

In a Phase II study of 35 patients with mature T-cell lymphomas of other subtypes with variable CD30 expression, ORR was 33% for PTCL-NOS and 54% for AITL, with CR rates of 14% and 38%, respectively. There was no correlation between the degree of CD30 expression and response in this trial.

Adverse events. In the Phase II registration study, grade 3 or greater neutropenia was the most common adverse event, occurring in 55% of patients; peripheral neuropathy occurred in 53% and anemia in 52%.

Grading and management of peripheral neuropathy is an integral part of therapeutic planning with brentuximab vedotin, and informs dose adjustments, treatment delays and discontinuations. The Total Neuropathy Score, which includes pinprick and vibration sensations, is a validated tool to measure sensory, autonomic and motor symptoms and may be helpful in the management of patients receiving brentuximab vedotin.[15]

Mogamulizumab (KW-0761) is a humanized antibody targeted against CCR4 (also designated CD194) with enhanced antibody-dependent cellular cytotoxicity. CCR4 is expressed in up to 65% of patients with PTCL, as well as in a subset of normal T cells, including type 2 helper T cells and regulatory T cells.

Efficacy and dosage. The registration trial that supported approval in Japan was a multicenter Phase II study in patients with relapsed or refractory ATLL, who received mogamulizumab intravenously at a dose of 1.0 mg/kg weekly for 4 weeks and then every 2 weeks.[7] Twenty-eight patients were enrolled, 52% with the acute form of the disease, 22% with the lymphoma presentation and 26% with chronic ATLL. The ORR was 50%, with a CR rate of 31%, and the drug was active at all disease sites.

A retrospective study in Japan reported outcomes from 77 patients with relapsed (23) or refractory (54) ATLL.[16] The ORR was 42%, with 18 CR and 15 PR. The median survival time from administration of mogamulizumab was 7.7 months.

A prospective study that compared mogamulizumab versus the investigator's choice of treatment of ATLL, conducted in the USA and Europe, reported best response rates of 28% and 8%, respectively.[17] Blinded independent review determined an ORR of 11%.

The activity of mogamulizumab in other PTCL subtypes has been explored in two studies.

- A European study enrolled 35 patients with relapsed PTCL, 11% of whom responded, with a PFS of 2 months.[18] The response rate was 13% in those with PTCL-NOS and 15% in those with AITL; no responses were seen in patients with ALCL.
- A Japanese study involving 38 patients reported a response rate of 35% (13 of 37), including five CRs. Median PFS was 3 months.[19] Responses were seen in patients with PTCL-NOS (19%) and AITL (50%), and in one patient with ALK⁻ ALCL.

Adverse events in the registration trial included infusion reactions in 89% of patients and skin rash in 63%. Of 14 patients with grade 2 or higher skin rash, 8 had a CR and 5 had a PR. Lymphopenia occurred in 96% of patients.

The most common side effects in the Japanese study were cytopenia, rash, pyrexia and infusion reactions. Almost half (22 of 51 patients) who received more than four doses of mogamulizumab had skin reactions. Interestingly, disease outcomes were superior in those patients who experienced a rash, as compared to patients with no skin reaction.

PI3K inhibitors

The phosphatidyl-inositol 3-kinase (PI3K) inhibitors have shown activity in both B- and T-cell malignancies.

Duvelisib (IPI-145) inhibits the gamma and delta subunits of PI3K. In a Phase I study of duvelisib, 25–100 mg daily, in patients with CTCL and PTCL (19 and 16 patients, respectively), the ORR was 50% in patients with relapsed and refractory PTCL, with 3 CR, and a median PFS of 8.3 months.[20] Adverse effects included elevated liver enzymes, cytopenia, skin rash and immune-mediated pneumonitis. Studies of duvelisib in combination with romidepsin and bortezomib are in progress.

Copanlisib (BAY-80-6946) is a PI3K alpha and delta inhibitor which showed activity in B-cell lymphomas and is approved by the FDA for the treatment of follicular B cell lymphoma. It is currently being evaluated in T-cell lymphomas.

Checkpoint inhibitors

Checkpoint inhibitors have shown therapeutic benefit in many types of cancer. They act at a crucial intersection between malignant cells and immune effector cells in the tumor microenvironment. PD-1 recognizes ligands such as PD-L1 on tumor cells, leading to evasion of the host immune response. Inhibitors of PD-1 and other immune-blocking epitopes such as CTLA-4 have shown promise and are approved for the treatment of a range of refractory malignancies.

Checkpoint inhibitors have yet to be investigated extensively in PTCL. Some partial responses were seen in five patients with PTCL treated with nivolumab in a Phase IB study.[21] ENKTCL appear to be particularly sensitive to checkpoint blockade. A study of seven patients with relapsed ENKTCL treated with pembrolizumab, 100 mg every 2 weeks, reported 2 CR and 2 PR, and response correlated with reduction in Epstein–Barr virus titers.[22]

Results in patients with ATLL associated with the HTLV-1 virus have been mixed, with some patients demonstrating disease progression.[23] Further studies are exploring the role of checkpoint inhibitors, alone and in combination, in patients with aggressive T-cell lymphomas.

Other novel agents

Alisertib is an inhibitor of Aurora A kinase, which is overexpressed in PTCL. A Phase II study of alisertib in 37 patients with relapsed and refractory PTCL reported an ORR of 30%.[24] A randomized Phase III trial compared alisertib, 50 mg daily for 7 days of a 21-day cycle, versus the investigator's choice of treatment (romidepsin, pralatrexate or gemcitabine) in 271 patients with relapsed or refractory PTCL. The ORR for alisertib was 33%, with PFS of 115 days, versus 104 days for the comparator arm. The ORRs in the comparator arm were 35% for gemcitabine (n = 8 of 23), 43% for pralatrexate (22 of 51 patients), and 61% for romidepsin (11 of 18 patients). Adverse events with alisertib included bone marrow suppression and diarrhea.[25]

Bendamustine is a bifunctional alkylating agent with chloroethylamine attached to a benzimidazole moiety. The Phase II BENTLY trial evaluated the activity of bendamustine, 120 mg/m², in 60 patients with relapsed or refractory PTCL.[26] The ORR was high but the DOR was short (3.5 months) and only 7% of patients had responses lasting a year.

Lenalidomide has anti-proliferative, anti-antiogenic and immunomodulatory effects across a range of hematologic malignancies, including demonstrable activity in relapsed PTCL. Several single-arm trials exploring lenalidomide, 25 mg per day for 21 consecutive days in 28-day cycles, reported response rates of 22–30% in heavily pretreated patients with AITL, ALCL or PTCL-NOS.[27] The DOR was 3–5 months, and there was no evidence of sustained benefit.

Lenalidomide in combination with romidepsin was explored in a Phase II trial in which romidepsin was administered at 8–14 mg/m² on days 1, 8 and 15, and lenalidomide at 15–25 mg/day for 21 consecutive days of a 28-day cycle. The response rate in patients with PTCL was 67%.[28]

Key points – treatment of relapsed and refractory PTCL

- Patients with relapsed and refractory PTCL who are not candidates for potentially curative allogeneic stem cell transplantation have poor outcomes with conventional chemotherapy regimens.
- A clinical trial should be regarded as the standard of care for patients with relapsed and refractory PTCL.
- Single-agent therapies and novel agents have demonstrated activity in PTCL. Although the duration of response is typically short, these are options for patients who are not eligible for stem cell transplantation.
- Histone deacetylase inhibitors are often active in patients with AITL because of epigenetic mutations.
- Brentuximab vedotin is highly active in ALCL and has demonstrated activity in CD30-expressing subsets of PTCL. Neurotoxicity is a frequent adverse event and requires careful monitoring.

Key references

1. Mak V, Hamm J, Chhanabhai M et al. Survival of patients with peripheral T-cell lymphoma after first relapse or progression: spectrum of disease and rare long-term survivors. *J Clin Oncol* 2013;31:1970–6.

2. Bellei M, Foss FM, Shustov AR et al. The outcome of peripheral T-cell lymphoma patients failing first-line therapy: a report from the prospective, International T-Cell Project. *Haematologica* 2018;103:1191–7.

3. O'Connor OA, Pro B, Pinter-Brown L et al. Pralatrexate in patients with relapsed or refractory peripheral T-cell lymphoma: results from the pivotal PROPEL study. *J Clin Oncol* 2011;29:1182–9.

4. Coiffier B, Pro B, Prince HM et al. Results from a pivotal, open-label, phase II study of romidepsin in relapsed or refractory peripheral T-cell lymphoma after prior systemic therapy. *J Clin Oncol* 2012;30:631–6.

5. O'Connor OA, Horwitz S, Masszi T et al. Belinostat in patients with relapsed or refractory peripheral T-cell lymphoma: results of the pivotal phase II BELIEF (CLN-19) study. *J Clin Oncol* 2015;33:2492–9.

6. Shi Y, Dong M, Hong X et al. Results from a multicenter, open-label, pivotal phase II study of chidamide in relapsed or refractory peripheral T-cell lymphoma. *Ann Oncol* 2015;26:1766–71.

7. Yamamoto K, Utsunomiya A, Tobinai K et al. Phase I study of KW-0761, a defucosylated humanized anti-CCR4 antibody, in relapsed patients with adult T-cell leukemia-lymphoma and peripheral T-cell lymphoma. *J Clin Oncol* 2010;28:1591–8.

8. Foss FM, Parker TL, Girardi M, Li A. Clinical activity of pralatrexate in patients with cutaneous T-cell lymphoma treated with varying doses of pralatrexate. *Clin Lymphoma Myeloma Leuk* 2018;18:e445–7.

9. Piekarz RL, Frye R, Prince HM et al. Phase 2 trial of romidepsin in patients with peripheral T-cell lymphoma. *Blood* 2011;117:5827–34.

10. Foss F, Pro B, Miles Prince H et al. Responses to romidepsin by line of therapy in patients with relapsed or refractory peripheral T-cell lymphoma. *Cancer Med* 2017;6: 36–44.

11. Foss F, Advani R, Duvic M et al. A Phase II trial of belinostat (PXD101) in patients with relapsed or refractory peripheral or cutaneous T-cell lymphoma. *Br J Haematol* 2015;168:811–19.

12. Bossard C, Dobay MP, Parrens M et al. Immunohistochemistry as a valuable tool to assess CD30 expression in peripheral T-cell lymphomas: high correlation with mRNA levels. *Blood* 2014;124:2983–6.

13. Horwitz S, O'Connor OA, Pro B et al. Brentuximab vedotin with chemotherapy for CD30-positive peripheral T-cell lymphoma (ECHELON-2): a global, double-blind, randomised, phase 3 trial. *Lancet* 2019;393:229–40.

14. Pro B, Advani R, Brice P et al. Brentuximab vedotin (SGN-35) in patients with relapsed or refractory systemic anaplastic large-cell lymphoma: results of a phase II study. *J Clin Oncol* 2012;30:2190–6.

15. Corbin ZA, Nguyen-Lin A, Li S et al. Characterization of the peripheral neuropathy associated with brentuximab vedotin treatment of mycosis fungoides and sezary syndrome. *J Neurooncol* 2017;132:439–46.

16. Sekine M, Kubuki Y, Kameda T et al. Effects of mogamulizumab in adult T-cell leukemia/lymphoma in clinical practice. *Eur J Haematol* 2017;98:501–7.

17. Phillips AA, Fields PA, Hermine O et al. Mogamulizumab versus investigator choice of chemotherapy regimen in relapsed/refractory adult T-cell leukemia/lymphoma. *Haematologica* 2019;104:993–1003.

18. Zinzani PL, Karlin L, Radford J et al. European phase II study of mogamulizumab, an anti-CCR4 monoclonal antibody, in relapsed/refractory peripheral T-cell lymphoma. *Haematologica* 2016;101:e407–10.

19. Ogura M, Ishida T, Hatake K et al. Multicenter phase II study of mogamulizumab (KW-0761), a defucosylated anti-cc chemokine receptor 4 antibody, in patients with relapsed peripheral T-cell lymphoma and cutaneous T-cell lymphoma. *J Clin Oncol* 2014;32:1157–63.

20. Horwitz SM, Koch R, Porcu P et al. Activity of the PI3K-δ,γ inhibitor duvelisib in a phase 1 trial and preclinical models of T-cell lymphoma. *Blood* 2018;131:888–98.

21. Lesokhin AM, Ansell SM, Armand P et al. Nivolumab in patients with relapsed or refractory hematologic malignancy: preliminary results of a Phase Ib study. *J Clin Oncol* 2016;34:2698–704.

22. Li X, Cheng Y, Zhang M et al. Activity of pembrolizumab in relapsed/refractory NK/T-cell lymphoma. *J Hematol Oncol* 2018;11:15.

23. Ratner L, Waldmann TA, Janakiram M, Brammer JE. Rapid progression of adult T-cell leukemia-lymphoma after PD-1 inhibitor therapy. *N Engl J Med* 2018;378:1947–8.

24. Barr PM, Li H, Spier C et al. Phase II Intergroup Trial of alisertib in relapsed and refractory peripheral T-cell lymphoma and transformed mycosis fungoides: SWOG 1108. *J Clin Oncol* 2015;33:2399–404.

25. O'Connor OA, Özcan M, Jacobsen ED et al. Randomized phase III study of alisertib or investigator's choice (selected single agent) in patients with relapsed or refractory peripheral T-cell lymphoma. *J Clin Oncol* 2019;37:613–23.

26. Damaj G, Gressin R, Bouabdallah K et al. Results from a prospective, open-label, phase II trial of bendamustine in refractory or relapsed T-cell lymphomas: the BENTLY trial. *J Clin Oncol* 2013;31:104–10.

27. Morschhauser F, Fitoussi O, Haioun C et al. A phase 2, multicentre, single-arm, open-label study to evaluate the safety and efficacy of single-agent lenalidomide (Revlimid) in subjects with relapsed or refractory peripheral T-cell non-Hodgkin lymphoma: the EXPECT trial. *Eur J Cancer* 2013;49:2869–76.

28. Broccoli A, Argnani L, Zinzani PL. Peripheral T-cell lymphomas: focusing on novel agents in relapsed and refractory disease. *Cancer Treat Rev* 2017;60:120–9.

7 Stem cell transplantation

Lohith Gowda MD MRCP (UK), Hematology and Bone Marrow Transplantation, Yale University School of Medicine, New Haven, CT, USA

The current standard of care for PTCL is anthracycline-based CHOP, followed by consolidation in first complete remission (CR1) with autologous stem cell transplantation (ASCT) in fit and eligible patients, given that remission tends to be short following induction chemotherapy.[1] According to the National Comprehensive Cancer Network guidelines, ASCT is recommended for all patients except those with ALK+ ALCL. Allogeneic stem cell transplantation (alloSCT) may be considered for patients with high-risk subtypes of PTCL (i.e. ENKTCL, ATLL and HSTCL).

The rarity and heterogeneity of PTCL have precluded a large randomized study to assess the best consolidation strategy (ASCT or alloSCT) after completing induction therapy, and studies comparing consolidation transplantation versus maintenance therapy have not been conducted. Prospective and retrospective Phase II studies are confounded by the highly selected populations of patients fit enough to tolerate transplantation and those in complete remission prior to transplant – a highly chemosensitive group. Retrospective series have not compared outcomes in patients who undergo transplant versus those who achieved similar responses but did not undergo transplant.

Trials conducted to date have been so heterogeneous that it is not yet possible to identify prognostic and risk factors to inform the decision to proceed to transplantation.

Autologous stem cell transplantation

Following induction chemotherapy to debulk disease burden, hematopoietic stem cells are harvested by apheresis and frozen. The patient then receives high-dose chemotherapy (HDT) to eradicate the residual malignant cell pool, but at the cost of partial or complete bone marrow ablation. The stored stem cells are then retransfused to replace the destroyed tissue and resume normal blood cell production. Autologous transplant allows rapid recovery of immune function, reducing the risk of infection during the immune-compromised period. In addition, the risk of graft versus host disease (GVHD) is low because the patient receives a transplant of their own cells.

Evidence for and against upfront ASCT. Studies in CR1 report progression-free survival (PFS) rates of 30–53% and overall survival (OS) rates of 34–73% for a range of histologically different PTCL subtypes. In intent-to-treat (ITT) studies, 40–73% of patients proceeded to transplant, while the remaining patients developed either progressive disease or comorbidities that precluded ASCT.

The NLG-T-01 study conducted by the Nordic Lymphoma Group explored ASCT in 160 patients with newly diagnosed PTCL (other than ALK+ ALCL).[2] Patients up to 60 years of age received three courses of biweekly CHOEP induction whereas older patients received standard CHOP because of reported toxicity with etoposide. Overall, 131 patients (82%) achieved a complete response (CR) or partial response (PR) at the end of induction; 25 (16%) had primary refractory disease. Among the responders, 115 (72%) proceeded to HDT with either BEAM or BEAC followed by ASCT: 90 were in CR 3 months after ASCT and 9 achieved PR.

In the longer term, 28 patients (18%) experienced disease relapse within 2 years and 11 (7%) patients experienced relapse beyond 2 years. OS at median follow-up of 5 years was 51%, and PFS was 44%. Five-year survival outcomes for different subtypes of PTCL are shown in Table 7.1. Treatment-related mortality (TRM) was 4% for the entire cohort.

TABLE 7.1

Five-year survival rates in the NLG-T-01 study of upfront autologous stem cell transplantation[2]

	Overall survival (%)	Progression-free survival (%)
ALK− ALCL	70	61
AITL	52	49
EATL	48	38
PTCL-NOS	47	38
Overall	51	44

Advanced age and bone marrow involvement were associated with inferior outcomes. The International Prognostic Index (IPI) score predicted OS in patients with AITL, and PFS in those with PTCL-NOS or AITL. ALCL histology and female sex were positive predictive variables.

Reimer and colleagues reported a dose-intensification study (n = 83) in which CHOP-based induction was followed by myeloablative cyclophosphamide/total body irradiation conditioning and ASCT.[3] Fifty-five of the patients (66%) proceeded to transplantation. Disease progression was the most frequent reason for not receiving ASCT. The overall response rate was 66% (56% CR; 8% PR%). Half of the patients (43; 52%) were alive at a median of 33 months' follow up. Three-year OS and PFS rates were 48% and 36%, respectively.

Han and colleagues reported a retrospective analysis of ASCT in 46 Chinese patients.[4] CR was achieved before transplant in 34 patients and PR in 12. The 5-year PFS and OS rates were 62% and 77%, respectively (median follow-up 37 months; range 6–176). In multivariate analysis, pretransplant CR was an independent risk factor for survival.

The US Center for International Blood and Marrow Transplantation Registry (CIBMTR), which collects data from US transplant centers, reported outcomes for T-cell lymphomas in 2013, based on 115 patients (median age 43 years at time of transplant). The 3-year PFS and OS rates for patients beyond CR1 were 42% and 53%, respectively.[5]

The COMPLETE study, which aimed to identify modern practice at large US academic centers, prospectively collected treatment and disease information for 499 patients with nodal PTCL.[6] A total of 213 achieved CR following frontline therapy; 64 (30%) went on to receive transplant (49 ASCT , 15 alloSCT), whereas 149 (70%) did not receive consolidation transplantation. Multivariate analysis showed that ASCT was associated with superior OS for patients who achieved CR.

Fossard and colleagues. In contrast to the studies above, this large multicenter retrospective study throws some doubt on the value or necessity of ASCT.[7] This study compared outcomes with and without ASCT in 269 patients (aged ≤ 65 years) with PTCL-NOS (n = 78), AITL (n = 123) or ALK+ ALCL (n = 68). CR was achieved with induction chemotherapy in 217 (81%) and PR in 52 (19%). Half the patients (n = 134) went on to ASCT (ITT). Comparison of the groups who did and did not receive transplant was based on a multivariate proportional hazard model, with propensity score matching to correct for sample selection bias. Neither method found a survival advantage in favor of ASCT, and no differences were identified between the groups in terms of response status, disease stage or risk category. Critics of this study point out the pitfalls of retrospective studies.

Allogeneic stem cell transplantation

Approximately 30% of patients have HLA-identical sibling donors for alloSCT; the remainder depend on matched unrelated or mismatched related/unrelated donors. In the US national marrow donor program, the probability of finding a donor can be as high as 70–75% for white patients but as low as 5–10% for some minority groups.[8] To address the shortage of donors for eligible patients, transplants using umbilical cord blood and haplo-identical transplants (>95% donor availability) have increasingly been used over the last decade, with encouraging results. Choosing the right graft for a patient is an important consideration.

In general, alloSCT at CR1 is preferred for the aggressive PTCLs – HSTCL, γδ-TCL, ATLL and ENKTCL. With this approach, donor T and natural killer (NK) cells exert a graft versus lymphoma (GVL) effect, regardless of whether the disease is chemosensitive or -refractory, although the former is associated with longer PFS. Following transplant, the donor T cells undergo thymic-dependent maturation, and a broad T-cell repertoire is achieved in the new host over 1–2 years. Until this process is complete, immune surveillance is conducted by graft-associated T cells (passenger lymphocytes), NK cells and the recipient's own T cells that survive conditioning and undergo homeostatic expansion.[9] Once the grafted T cells have attained a wide range of competence, the risk of relapse or infections is reduced, highlighting the significance of GVL and explaining why late relapse (beyond 1–2 years) is rare (in most studies, survival curves plateau by 2 years).

AlloSCT in refractory/relapsed disease. As with ASCT, clinical practice has been informed by retrospective and registry-based studies in the absence of randomized studies. Le Gouill and colleagues reported data from 77 patients in a French registry;[10] at the time of transplant, 40% of patients were in CR, 30% were in PR and 30% had stable, progressive or refractory disease. The 5-year PFS and OS rates were 53% and 57%, respectively, and were influenced by disease status at the time of transplant. Survival rates in patients with different histologic subtypes are shown in Table 7.2. An OS rate of 29% was seen in the chemoresistant population. Patients who did not achieve CR after alloSCT died within the 10 months' follow-up. The 5-year TRM rate was 33%, largely associated with the use of mismatched donors.

Based on anecdotal reports of high TRM (30%) with MAC induction chemotherapy, Corradini evaluated reduced-intensity conditioning (RIC) followed by alloSCT (n = 17; median age at transplant 41 years).[11] Fifteen patients had relapsed disease and two had primary refractory disease. Three-year PFS and OS rates were estimated at 81% and 64%, respectively, with a low non-relapse mortality (NRM) rate of 6%. In two patients who had disease relapse after transplantation, a response was induced by the infusion of donor lymphocytes, confirming a GVL effect.

The CIBMTR study has also published outcomes from a large cohort of heavily pretreated patients (n = 126; median age at transplant, 38 years).[5] GVL was seen across different histologic subtypes. The survival and NRM rates are shown in Table 7.3.

In summary, alloSCT offers long-term disease control in 30–55% of patients with relapsed/refractory PTCL but is associated with NRM rates of 12–36%. NRM rates are expected to be improved through

TABLE 7.2

Five-year survival rates in 77 patients undergoing allogeneic stem cell transplantation[10]

PTCL subtype	Overall survival (%)	Progression-free survival (%)
AITL	80	80
PTCL-NOS	58	63
ALCL	48	55
Miscellaneous subgroups	33	Not reported

TABLE 7.3

Survival rates and non-relapse mortality following alloSCT in the CIBMTR study

	Progression-free survival rate (%)	Overall survival rate (%)	1-/3-year non-relapse mortality rates (%)
ALCL	35	41	29/31
PTCL	33	42	28/29
AITL	67	83	8/8

high-resolution donor typing and improvements in antimicrobial and GVHD prophylaxis.

AlloSCT at first remission. Data on alloSCT in CR1 are limited. Loirat and colleagues evaluated the feasibility of upfront alloSCT in advanced PTCL.[12] In this ITT study, 29 of 49 patients (60%) proceeded to allograft. One- and 2-year OS rates after transplant were 76% and 72.5%, respectively and the TRM at 1 year was 8.2%. For patients who did not proceed to alloSCT, 2-year PFS was less than 30%.

Corradini and colleagues have also reported findings from a prospective study of 64 patients who received chemoimmunotherapy followed by ASCT (n = 14) or alloSCT (n = 23) depending on donor availability following a conditioning regimen of fludarabine, cyclophosphamide and thiotepa.[13] At the time of reporting, 16 of 23 patients were in CR, and seven had died (four from disease; three from toxicity).

The benefits with alloSCT in CR1 to potentially achieve a long-term remission need to be balanced against the short- and long-term toxicity and mortality risk associated with the procedure. Treatment should be informed by discussion and the preferences of the patient.

AlloSCT for specific PTCL subtypes

ATLL. Given the association of ATLL with human T-cell lymphotropic virus 1 (HTLV-1), outcomes data are primarily from Japanese patients and patients of Caribbean descent living in the west. A large Japanese registry study reported median OS following alloSCT of 9.9 months and a 3-year OS rate of 36%.[14] Survival was similar with

MAC and RIC, although there was a trend towards slightly better survival with RIC. Multivariate analysis showed that older age, male sex, absence of CR, poor performance status and unrelated donor grafts were associated with worse OS.

A single center US study of 53 patients of Caribbean descent[15] reported a response rate of 32% with anthracycline-based therapy. Five patients underwent alloSCT, and two achieved CR even though pretransplant status had confirmed residual or relapsed phenotype. One patient whose disease relapsed after alloSCT responded to immunosuppression withdrawal but ultimately succumbed to GVHD.

These studies suggest that responses to induction therapy are poor in both Japanese and Caribbean patients with ATLL. Hence, alloSCT should be offered for fit and eligible patients in CR1. A lack of targeted agents has prompted clinicians to also consider alloSCT in patients with PR, with durable response seen in some.

ENKTCL. Murashige and colleagues reported a study of 28 patients in Japan with predominantly ENKTCL (n = 22) who underwent alloSCT: 2-year PFS and OS rates were 34% and 40%, respectively.[16] Kanate and colleagues reported a US study (n = 82) of primarily Caucasian patients (66%), with a smaller cohort of Asian descent (16%). At the time of transplant, 45% of patients were in CR, 30% were in PR and 12% had chemorefractory disease. Most patients received a peripheral blood graft (89%), had a matched sibling donor (61%) and received RIC (59%). The 3-year OS and PFS rates were 34% and 28%, respectively; no relapses were seen 2 years after transplant.[17]

Patients with aggressive NK leukemia also experience similarly poor outcomes, with estimated 2-year OS and PFS rates of 24% and 20%, respectively.[18]

HSTCL is generally associated with poor outcomes.[19] Published literature are limited because of the rarity of the disease although a systematic review of transplant outcomes has been reported.[20] A total of 54 patients were identified, with a median age at transplantation of 34 years; 94% had stage IV disease. At the time of alloSCT, 41% and 43% were in CR and PR, respectively and 16% had progressive disease. Most (70%) received MAC; the remainder received RIC. Post-transplant outcomes data were available for 44 patients. Median PFS and OS were 18 months and 64 months, respectively, and 3-year PFS and OS rates were estimated at 42% and 56%, respectively. Active disease at the time of transplant was not associated with poor outcomes, which suggests that GVL can, to some extent, overcome chemoresistance. The European Society for Blood and Marrow Transplantation reported outcomes for 18 patients who underwent alloSCT:[21] at a median follow up of 3 years, 2 patients had disease relapse post-transplant and the 3-year PFS was 48%.

Allogeneic versus autologous transplant

A 2016 study retrospectively compared ASCT and alloSCT in 60 patients with high-risk PTCL (IPI score ≥ 3), 22 with PTCL-NOS, 22 with ALK⁻ ALCL and 16 with AITL.[22] Before transplant, 40 patients were in CR and 2 were in PR. Twenty-one patients received alloSCT and 39 received ASCT (a higher proportion of patients in CR received ASCT). Survival outcomes based on Kaplan–Meier analysis at a median follow-up of 39 months (range 1–96) were similar between the two groups (Table 7.4). However, there were fewer relapses following alloSCT and the cumulative recurrence rate was also lower (but not significant). This study demonstrates the potential of GVL in patients with high-risk PTCL even if CR or PR is not achieved before transplant.

Complications of transplant

Short-term complications. Immediate post-transplant complications include cytopenia and mucosal aberration and are similar with ASCT and alloSCT. Deficiencies in cellular immunity post-transplant may lead to viral or fungal infection, especially in the setting of

TABLE 7.4

Five-year outcomes with autologous and allogeneic stem cell transplantation

	Autologous	Allogeneic
Progression-free survival	61%	60%
Overall survival	62%	61%
Cumulative transplant-related mortality	0%	16.5%
Number of relapses	7	2
Cumulative recurrence rate	37.2%	10.1%

immunosuppression. The routine use of gram-negative prophylaxis has reduced infectious complications from gut transmigration. Use of prophylactic antivirals has also reduced associated mortality.

Graft versus host disease is an important reason for the high TRM with alloSCT compared with ASCT. The incidence of all-grade acute GVHD is 20–50% with HLA-matched siblings and 20–70% for unrelated HLA-mismatched donors. Rates of chronic GVHD can be about 50% with commonly used calcineurin-based prophylaxis. Other than steroids, there are no good second-line drugs for the management of acute or chronic GVHD, and fewer than 20% of patients with steroid-refractory disease survive beyond 1 year.[9] Ongoing trials are evaluating novel mechanistic-based drugs, therapies targeting regulatory T cells, selective $\alpha\beta$ T-cell depletion and infusion of genetically engineered T cells with a caspase-based suicide switch that can be used to abrogate alloreactive T-cell function without compromising immune surveillance.

Secondary neoplasms are a well-known complication in transplant survivors, attributable to the mutagenic chemoradiotherapy and immunosuppressants used in the transplant setting. Solid organ tumors (0.7–1.7%), leukemias/myelodysplastic syndrome (1–4.7%) and post-transplant lymphoproliferative disorders (0.1%) are all well described in the transplant literature.[23] The risk of neoplasms appears to peak 5 years after transplant. Establishment of long-term survivor clinics to monitor for these developments would enable early diagnosis and timely therapeutic intervention.

Disease recurrence is still one of the common causes of treatment failure after transplant. To decrease post-transplant relapse, targeted agents with conditioning regimens, dose-modulation of preparative regimens and post-transplant maintenance strategies (e.g. brentuximab vedotin, checkpoint inhibitors, romidepsin) are being explored, with encouraging preliminary results. However, the reduction in the risk of disease relapse with such approaches needs to be balanced against potential toxicity, and the widespread use of drug maintenance for all transplant recipients needs to be explored. Better understanding of disease biology may change this approach.

Future directions

The potential of GVL following stem cell transplantation to decrease relapse rates compared with other contemporary treatment modalities in the management of PTCL has been clearly demonstrated. However, disease relapse is still the most common cause of treatment failure. Improving the quality of the pretransplant response holds significant promise in prolonging post-transplant survival, and maintenance with less toxic pharmacologic agents may also offer a way to reduce relapse rates.

Key points – stem cell transplantation

- Autologous stem cell transplant (ASCT) as a consolidation strategy is an option for patients who achieve a complete response with front-line chemotherapy.
- Phase II studies have shown that about 40% of patients who undergo ASCT at first remission are disease free at 5 years.
- Allogeneic stem cell transplantation (alloSCT) provides long-term disease control in patients with relapsed or refractory PTCL and as a front-line consolidation for patients with more aggressive PTCL subtypes.
- Complications from alloSCT include serious infections resulting from immune suppression, and chronic graft versus host disease.
- In a randomized study, outcomes were similar with upfront ASCT and alloSCT, with more patients in the autologous arm relapsing and more in the allogeneic arm experiencing transplant-related morbidity and mortality.

Key references

1. Parrilla Castellar ER, Jaffe ES, Said JW et al. ALK-negative anaplastic large cell lymphoma is a genetically heterogeneous disease with widely disparate clinical outcomes. *Blood* 2014;124:1473–80.

2. d'Amore F, Relander T, Lauritzsen GF et al. Up-front autologous stem-cell transplantation in peripheral T-cell lymphoma: NLG-T-01. *J Clin Oncol* 2012;30:3093–9.

3. Reimer P, Rudiger T, Geissinger E et al. Autologous stem-cell transplantation as first-line therapy in peripheral T-cell lymphomas: results of a prospective multicenter study. *J Clin Oncol* 2009;27:106–13.

4. Han X, Zhang W, Zhou D et al. Autologous stem cell transplantation as frontline strategy for peripheral T-cell lymphoma: a single-centre experience. *J Int Med Res* 2017; 45:290–302.

5. Smith SM, Burns LJ, van Besien K et al. Hematopoietic cell transplantation for systemic mature T-cell non-Hodgkin lymphoma. *J Clin Oncol* 2013;31:3100–9.

6. Carson KR, Horwitz SM, Pinter-Brown LC et al. A prospective cohort study of patients with peripheral T-cell lymphoma in the United States. *Cancer* 2017;123:1174–83.

7. Fossard G, Broussais F, Coelho I et al. Role of up-front autologous stem-cell transplantation in peripheral T-cell lymphoma for patients in response after induction: an analysis of patients from LYSA centers. *Ann Oncol* 2018;29:715–23.

8. Gragert L, Eapen M, Williams E et al. HLA match likelihoods for hematopoietic stem-cell grafts in the U.S. registry. *N Engl J Med* 2014;371:339–48.

9. Mehta RS, Rezvani K. Immune reconstitution post allogeneic transplant and the impact of immune recovery on the risk of infection. *Virulence* 2016;7:901–16.

10. Le Gouill S, Milpied N, Buzyn A et al. Graft-versus-lymphoma effect for aggressive T-cell lymphomas in adults: a study by the Societe Francaise de Greffe de Moelle et de Therapie Cellulaire. *J Clin Oncol* 2008;26:2264–71.

11. Corradini P, Dodero A, Zallio F et al. Graft-versus-lymphoma effect in relapsed peripheral T-cell non-Hodgkin's lymphomas after reduced-intensity conditioning followed by allogeneic transplantation of hematopoietic cells. *J Clin Oncol* 2004;22:2172–6.

12. Loirat M, Chevallier P, Leux C et al. Upfront allogeneic stem-cell transplantation for patients with nonlocalized untreated peripheral T-cell lymphoma: an intention-to-treat analysis from a single center. *Ann Oncol* 2015;26:386–92.

13. Corradini P, Vitolo U, Rambaldi A et al. Intensified chemo-immunotherapy including up-front autologous or allogeneic stem cell transplantation (SCT) for young patients with newly diagnosed peripheral T-cell lymphomas: final results of a phase II multicenter prospective clinical trial. *Blood* 2012;120:abstract 1984.

14. Ishida T, Hishizawa M, Kato K et al. Allogeneic hematopoietic stem cell transplantation for adult T-cell leukemia-lymphoma with special emphasis on preconditioning regimen: a nationwide retrospective study. *Blood* 2012;120:1734–41.

15. Zell M, Assal A, Derman O et al. Adult T-cell leukemia/lymphoma in the Caribbean cohort is a distinct clinical entity with dismal response to conventional chemotherapy. *Oncotarget* 2016;7:51 981–90.

16. Murashige N, Kami M, Kishi Y et al. Allogeneic haematopoietic stem cell transplantation as a promising treatment for natural killer-cell neoplasms. *Br J Haematol* 2005;130:561–7.

17. Kanate AS, DiGilio A, Ahn KW et al. Allogeneic haematopoietic cell transplantation for extranodal natural killer/T-cell lymphoma, nasal type: a CIBMTR analysis. *Br J Haematol* 2018;182:916–20.

18. Hamadani M, Kanate AS, DiGilio A et al. Allogeneic hematopoietic cell transplantation for aggressive NK cell leukemia. A Center for International Blood and Marrow Transplant Research analysis. *Biol Blood Marrow Transplant* 2017;23: 853–6.

19. Gowda L, Foss F. Hepatosplenic T-cell lymphomas. *Cancer Treat Res* 2019;176:185–93.

20. Rashidi A, Cashen AF. Outcomes of allogeneic stem cell transplantation in hepatosplenic T-cell lymphoma. *Blood Cancer J* 2015;5:e318.

21. Tanase A, Schmitz N, Stein H et al. Allogeneic and autologous stem cell transplantation for hepatosplenic T-cell lymphoma: a retrospective study of the EBMT Lymphoma Working Party. *Leukemia* 2015;29:686–8.

22. Huang H, Wang Q, Jin Z et al. A comparison study between allogeneic and autologous hematopoietic stem cell transplant for high-risk peripheral T-cell lymphomas. *Blood* 2016;128:5845.

23. Burns LJ. Late effects after autologous hematopoietic cell transplantation. *Biol Blood Marrow Transplant* 2009;15:21–4.

8 Research directions

Advances in molecular technologies are now making it possible to identify PTCL cohorts with shared molecular dependencies that span conventional histologic categories, enabling significant progress in our understanding of pathobiology across PTCL subtypes. This should, in turn, aid the development of novel precise mechanistic-based treatment strategies.

Tissue-based molecular studies

Next-generation sequencing (NGS) is a high-throughput method for detecting aberrations in DNA sequences: it can be used to interrogate a panel of specific genes (targeted), all coding regions of the genome (whole-exome sequencing; WES) or the entire genome (whole-genome sequencing; WGS). NGS research studies have identified distinct mutational signatures in AITL and Tfh-related lymphomas, and recurrent mutations in other PTCL subtypes (see Chapter 2). However, most studies have used targeted NGS or WES, providing only a limited view of the PTCL genome. Increasingly affordable sequencing platforms and improved bioinformatic pipelines will allow more PTCL cases to be interrogated by WGS, which should provide new mechanistic insights into the disease.

Integrated multiomic analysis. The biology of PTCL is likely to extend beyond aberrations in the genetic sequence. Transcriptomic, epigenetic, methylation and metabolomic programs are likely to be key cellular drivers of PTCL. The integration of sequencing data with multiomic analysis is likely to be critical in identifying vulnerabilities for drug targeting. Alternative molecular approaches can map genome-wide chromatin accessibility, DNA-bound proteins such as enhancers, and methylated cytosine residues. Such analysis will be particularly relevant for PTCL cases in which current sequencing strategies do not detect a recurrent mutation.

Challenges to molecular studies. NGS studies, especially WES or WGS approaches, require adequate quality and quantity of tissue to produce robust data. Patients with PTCL are often unwell at presentation and frequently require urgent therapy, resulting in the use of needle biopsies (rather than surgical excision biopsy), which yield limited samples. Some subtypes of PTCL, particularly AITL, are characterized by a heavy stromal infiltrate with low tumor burden, rendering bulk sequencing relatively insensitive. Moreover, studies in other cancers have demonstrated significant intratumor heterogeneity, suggesting that single-site biopsies may fail to capture the global tumor mutational composition, representing a major barrier to genomic-driven treatment strategies.

Blood-based sequencing assays

A potential solution to many of the challenges of tissue-based molecular studies is to use peripheral blood as a source of tumor DNA. Tumor DNA may be released into the circulation by dying cancer cells, or actively secreted. Circulating tumor DNA (ctDNA) offers a non-invasive way to determine tissue mutational status, assess global tumor heterogeneity and track tumor evolution in real time through serial sampling.[1,2] Increasing evidence supports the use of ctDNA in solid malignancies, and a recent study showed that ctDNA can predict clinical outcomes in aggressive B-cell lymphoma[3] and Hodgkin lymphoma.[4] The use of ctDNA in PTCL is being studied in several countries.

Single cell analysis

Bulk analysis generates an average profile of the whole cell population, including malignant and non-malignant cells, which does not adequately capture the complexity of a tumor and risks missing treatment-resistant subclones that will ultimately germinate relapse. However, technological developments enabling single cell analysis are allowing researchers to deconvolute bulk tumors and analyze cancers with greater resolution and accuracy (Figure 8.1). Single cell RNA and DNA sequencing can determine cancer evolution, provide insight into tumor heterogeneity and segregate and characterize stromal cells. Given that bulk sequencing of PTCL cases to date has been relatively insensitive, single cell analysis is likely to significantly advance our understanding of PTCL biology.

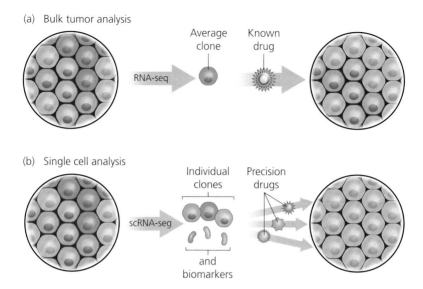

Figure 8.1 (a) Bulk tumor analysis mostly reflects dominant populations and averages data across various cancer subclones. Treatment chosen based on this information may prove ineffective as resistant subclones expand. (b) Single cell (sc) analysis can characterize individual subclones which can then be targeted using tailored drug combinations to eradicate malignant clones. RNA-seq, whole transcriptome shotgun sequencing.

Preclinical models

Advances in the treatment of PTCL have been significantly hampered by the paucity of relevant preclinical models. Only a relatively small number of PTCL cell lines are available, many of which are poorly characterized and are of limited value to preclinical testing. There is also a lack of genetically engineered mouse models that faithfully reflect human PTCL. Recent initiatives generating patient-derived xenograft PTCL models[5] may facilitate discoveries into PTCL biology and the development of novel treatment strategies.

Novel treatment strategies

A plethora of new drugs are being developed, including monoclonal antibodies against T-cell receptors, cytokines, and chemokines, small molecular inhibitors that target key T-cell pathways, and agents that reverse epigenetic dysregulation. It is unlikely that any single drug will be equally effective across all PTCL subtypes but a stratified approach may increase the likelihood of demonstrating a clear benefit in a subtype of PTCL, as illustrated in Figure 8.1. Disease rarity poses significant challenges, however. International collaboration, for example through the International Rare Cancer Initiative, will be essential to deliver practice-changing clinical trials for specific PTCL subtypes.

Chimeric antigen receptor T-cell therapy represents a novel treatment strategy that may prove transformative across PTCL subtypes, as in other hematologic malignancies. Peripheral blood T cells apheresed from patients are engineered to express a modified antigen receptor that recognizes a cancer target (Figure 8.2). They are then reinfused. Upon engagement with the target cell, activation of CAR T cells triggers cytotoxicity of the cancer cell. This process is illustrated in Figure 8.3.

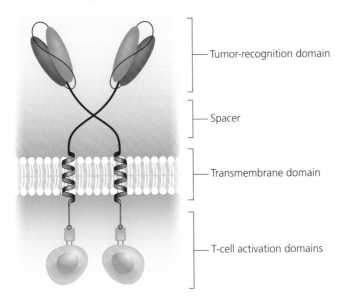

Tumor-recognition domain

Spacer

Transmembrane domain

T-cell activation domains

Figure 8.2 Chimeric antigen receptors (CARs) are membrane-bound proteins in which the tumor-recognition ability of an antibody is combined with naturally occurring T-cell activation mechanisms

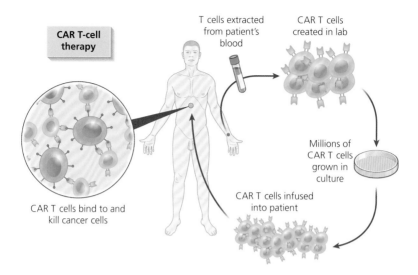

Figure 8.3 Chimeric antigen receptor (CAR) T-cell therapy.

CAR T cells have been developed for CD4, CD5, CD7 and CD30. However, some of these pan T-cell markers risk causing profound immunosuppression. An alternative approach is to develop CAR products against the T-cell receptor beta chain (TCRB). Peripheral T cells express two isoforms, TCRB1 and TCRB2, broadly evenly, but PTCL is clonally either TCRB1 or TCRB2. CAR products against these TCRB isoforms would therefore ensure that approximately half of the normal T-cell repertoire is preserved.[6]

Whilst promising, CAR T products are associated with significant toxicity, including cytokine release syndrome and neurotoxicity, and patients are at risk of rapid disease progression whilst awaiting CAR T-cell reinfusion. There is also uncertainty about tumor escape mechanisms.

Current research in specific PTCL subtypes
AITL and Tfh-related lymphomas. The recognition of a shared follicular helper T cell (Tfh) ontogeny provides a strong rationale for precision medicine,[7] and many novel drugs target key Tfh pathways (Table 8.1). Current studies are investigating novel therapies as monotherapies or in combination with other treatments, including

TABLE 8.1

Drugs in development for AITL and Tfh-related lymphomas

Drug	Class	Target	Rationale
Enasidenib	Small molecule	IDH2	Mutations in *IDH2*
Azacitidine	Hypomethylating agent	Epigenome	Mutations in *IDH2, TET2, DNMT3A*
Romidepsin Belinostat	HDAC inhibitors	Epigenome	
Duvelisib	Small molecules	PI3K	Mutations in TCR pathways
Ibrutinib (ONO-7790500)	Small molecules	ITK	
Abatacept	Monoclonal antibodies	CD80	Tfh-related pathway
Nivolumab Pembrolizumab		PD-1	
MEDI-570		ICOS	
VX5		CXCL13	

HDAC, histone deacetylase; TCR, T cell receptor; Tfh, follicular T helper cell. Molecular targets are defined in the list of abbreviations (page 4).
Adapted from Ahearne et al., 2014.[7]

azacytidine, phosphatidyl-inositol 3-kinase inhibitors, histidine deacetylase inhibitors and checkpoint inhibitors (see pages 64–73).

AITL has also been included alongside other cancers characterized by recurrent *IDH2* mutations (glioblastoma and acute myeloid leukemia) in a basket study assessing the isocitrate dehydrogenase 2 inhibitor enasidenib (NCT02273739).

PTCL-NOS. Up to a third of PTCL-NOS cases have mutations in the histone modifier gene,[3] suggesting that epigenetic targeting may have a role beyond Tfh lymphomas. A recent study has provided further support for two major biological and prognostic subgroups based on cell of origin: PTCL-GATA-3 and PTCL-TBX21 (see page 21). PTCL-GATA-3 showed a high proportion of alterations in the TP53 pathway and *STAT3/MYC* gains, whereas PTCL-TBX21 is characterized by *TET2* mutations and deletion of NF-κB pathway regulators.[8] Alternatively, PTCL-NOS can be divided from B cells and dendritic cells by microenvironmental signatures. These different PTCL-NOS signatures need to be tested in prospective clinical trials before they can be used to stratify patients in clinical practice.

ALCL. Studies are currently exploring the efficacy of crizotinib, an oral tyrosine kinase inhibitor, in blocking the oncogenic signals that derive from chromosomal translocations involving ALK. Early data suggest that crizotinib induces high response rates and is well tolerated.

Following the success with the targeted immunotoxin brentuximab vedotin in ALCL (see page 54), bispecific antibodies that bind CD30 and engage innate immune cells via CD16A, leading to lymphoma cell lysis, have been developed (Figure 8.4).

Both ALK+ and ALK− ALCL are characterized by *JAK-STAT* dysregulation, generating interest in the use of JAK inhibitors.

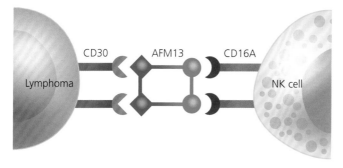

Figure 8.4 Bispecific antibodies that engage both CD16A expressed on natural killer (NK) cells and CD30 expressed on lymphoma cells are undergoing clinical testing. Bringing NK cells into close proximity with CD30-expressing lymphoma cells leads to NK cell activation, release of cytotoxic chemicals and lymphoma cell death.

EATL. The cell of origin has been identified as an intraepithelial innate lymphoid cell, a recently described heterogeneous immune subset. This insight is likely to precipitate further research and identify new drug targets. Interleukin (IL)-15 has been reported as a central player in lymphomagenesis,[9,10] and anti-IL15 monoclonal antibodies are being developed for refractory celiac disease and EATL (e.g. AMG-714).

NK cell malignancies largely express CD38, prompting evaluation of the CD38-directed antibody daratumumab (approved for the treatment of multiple myeloma) for ENKTCL. Immunogenic Epstein–Barr virus antigens (e.g. LMP1/2) are expressed heterogeneously in ENKTCL tissue and are a promising target for donor-derived[11] or engineered autologous cytotoxic T cells.[12]

Key points – research directions

- Next-generation sequencing has identified distinct DNA mutations in AITL and Tfh-related lymphomas, and recurrent mutations in other PTCL subtypes. Whole-genome studies should provide further insight across all PTCL subtypes.
- The integration of gene sequencing and multiomic analysis should help to identify vulnerabilities beyond aberrations of genetic sequences for drug targeting.
- The use of needle biopsies in patients with PTCL yield limits samples for molecular studies. However, circulating tumor DNA from peripheral blood may be an alternative.
- Patient-derived xenograft PTCL models may facilitate the development of new treatments and increase our understanding of PTCL biology.
- Given the high rates of chemoresistance and poor clinical outcomes for most patients with PTCL, novel precision medicine strategies are needed. A plethora of new drugs is in development, including monoclonal antibodies against T-cell receptors, cytokines and chemokines, small-molecule inhibitors, and agents that reverse epigenetic dysregulation.

Key references

1. Abbosh C, Birkbak NJ, Wilson GA et al. Phylogenetic ctDNA analysis depicts early-stage lung cancer evolution. *Nature* 2017;545:446–51.

2. Murtaza M, Dawson SJ, Pogrebniak K et al. Multifocal clonal evolution characterized using circulating tumour DNA in a case of metastatic breast cancer. *Nat Commun* 2015;6:8760.

3. Kurtz DM, Scherer F, Jin MC et al. Circulating tumor DNA measurements as early outcome predictors in diffuse large B-cell lymphoma. *J Clin Oncol* 2018; 36:2845–53.

4. Spina V, Bruscaggin A, Cuccaro A et al. Circulating tumor DNA reveals genetics, clonal evolution, and residual disease in classical Hodgkin lymphoma. *Blood* 2018;131:2413–25.

5. Ng SY, Yoshida N, Christie AL et al. Targetable vulnerabilities in T- and NK-cell lymphomas identified through preclinical models. *Nat Commun* 2018;9:2024.

6. Maciocia PM, Wawrzyniecka PA, Philip B et al. Targeting the T cell receptor beta-chain constant region for immunotherapy of T cell malignancies. *Nat Med* 2017;23: 1416–23.

7. Ahearne MJ, Allchin RL, Fox CP, Wagner SD. Follicular helper T-cells: expanding roles in T-cell lymphoma and targets for treatment. *Br J Haematol* 2014; 166:326–35.

8. Heavican TB, Bouska A, Yu J et al. Genetic drivers of oncogenic pathways in molecular subgroups of peripheral T-cell lymphoma. *Blood* 2019;133:1664–76.

9. Kooy-Winkelaar YM, Bouwer D, Janssen GM et al. CD4 T-cell cytokines synergize to induce proliferation of malignant and nonmalignant innate intraepithelial lymphocytes. *Proc Natl Acad Sci USA* 2017;114:E980–9.

10. Ettersperger J, Montcuquet N, Malamut G et al. Interleukin-15-dependent T-cell-like innate intraepithelial lymphocytes develop in the intestine and transform into lymphomas in celiac disease. *Immunity* 2016;45:610–25.

11. Vickers MA, Wilkie GM, Robinson N et al. Establishment and operation of a Good Manufacturing Practice-compliant allogeneic Epstein–Barr virus (EBV)-specific cytotoxic cell bank for the treatment of EBV-associated lymphoproliferative disease. *Br J Haematol* 2014;167:402–10.

12. Bollard CM, Gottschalk S, Torrano V et al. Sustained complete responses in patients with lymphoma receiving autologous cytotoxic T lymphocytes targeting Epstein-Barr virus latent membrane proteins. *J Clin Oncol* 2014;32:798–808.

Useful resources

UK

Lymphoma action
Helpline: 0808 808 5555
information@lymphoma-action.org.uk
lymphoma-action.org.uk

USA

Leukemia & Lymphoma Society
Toll-free: 1 800 955 4572
www.lls.org

Lymphoma Research Foundation
Helpline: 1 800 500 9976
helpline@lymphoma.org
www.lymphoma.org

T-cell Leukemia Lymphoma Foundation
Tel: 1 206 661 2253
info@tcllfoundation.org
www.tcllfoundation.org

International

Lymphoma Canada
Toll-free: +1 866 659 5556
info@lymphoma.ca
www.lymphoma.ca

Lymphoma Australia
Tel: +64 (0)7 3030 5050
enquiries@lymphoma.org.au
www.lymphoma.org.au

Leukemia & Lymphoma Society (Canada)
Tel: +1 888 557 7177
www.leukemia-lymphoma.org

Useful websites

Cancer Research UK
www.cancerresearchuk.org

T-cell Project 2.0
www.tcellproject2.org

Index